Humdinger!

noun:
an extraordinary
person or event

Stephanie and Paula are talking to you…visit their
YouTube…on the Welcome page …just click and you're there.

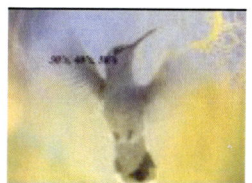

Go to **www.beataneurysmandleukemia.com**…

We're with you Providence.
You saved my life!
Stephanie I Heskins

Paula Snaman

Humdinger!

noun:
an extraordinary
person or event

Stephanie Ione Haskins
Paula Lanier Seaman

FOREWORD BY
DR. TERRY BERGESON

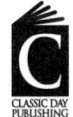

CLASSIC DAY
PUBLISHING

Seattle, Washington
Portland, Oregon
Denver, Colorado
Vancouver, B.C.
Scottsdale, Arizona
Minneapolis, Minnesota

ISBN: 978-1-59849-115-9
Library of Congress Control Number: 2011927619

Printed in the United States of America

Photographs: Kristin Zwiers
Design: Soundview Design Studio

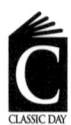

Classic Day Publishing
2925 Fairview Avenue East
Seattle, Washington 98102
877-728-8837
www.classicdaypub.com

Dedication

This book is dedicated to my very best friend in this world, Mary Heck, who is truly a believer. I first met her when she came to see me in February 2007 at Harborview. She truly understood me despite my tremendous difficulty communicating.

Her belief in me gave me the hope that through sharing my story I could actually make a difference for others.

She has stood by me every single step of the way – through many ups and downs. Without her support, wisdom, skills, humor, and understanding this book would not have been written and completed.

She is indeed a believer and she has made me one too. If we all believe we can stand together, we can, and if we do, we will win.

Contents

Foreword

BY TERRY BERGESON

Currently-Executive Director San Francisco School Alliance
Previously-Washington State Superintendent of Public Instruction

Humdinger! *noun: "An Extraordinary Person or Event"* is a story of life-threatening events and triumph over death and despair. The book is simple and direct, but it has a profound impact. If you are like me, once you pick it up, you won't be able to stop reading until the end, and you will be the better for it.

Stephanie Haskins and Paula Seaman are two of the most inspiring people I have ever met. Their story takes you through a totally unexpected personal journey of fear and courage and determination. It chronicles an amazing odyssey of their love of life and for each other and for the people who helped them along the way from February of 2007 until April of 2010 and beyond.

It is the story of Stephanie, a powerful woman with a mission for kids and public schools a trusted leader, articulate, highly skilled, passionate, and fiercely determined—a woman whose life was about making schools work for students and the educators who served them. Stephanie turned around the most struggling schools and brought joy and hope to the children and adults with whom she worked. Then suddenly a brain aneurysm struck her down.

She lost control of everything that made her who she was except for the inner spirit that drove her life.

It is also the story of Paula, a gifted, vibrant, and feisty educator in her own right and the woman who loved Stephanie deeply and unconditionally enough to support her when she was suddenly totally vulnerable. She was her trusted partner every single day through a three-and-a-half year medical ordeal that by all counts should have taken Stephanie's life.

It is also about the loving friends who supported Stephanie and Paula and were personally transformed by their courage and determination as they fought together for Stephanie's life and dignity. It's about the physicians and other medical personnel who had the empathy to recognize the startling strength of Stephanie's determination to survive her brutal illnesses and the power of Paula's love and courage to help her. They had the faith to keep treating her to the best of their ability in the face of daunting odds.

Finally, for me, as a fellow educator and a colleague and friend of these two incredible women, this story is a triumph of the human spirit and the human mind. The brain aneurysm and leukemia that attacked Stephanie robbed her temporarily of the intellectual and physical assets that were central to her life. She and Paula fought individually and as a team to win back Stephanie's life and dignity. As she won back herself, Stephanie also found peace and deeper wisdom. She and Paula are building a new life, but they will always be both teachers and helpers. So now they have given us this book to help countless others to find their way.

Paula's Story

◆ ◆ ◆

CHAPTER 1

Decision

February 9, 2007, was the night I had to make a life-or-death decision. I couldn't believe I would ever have to make a decision of this magnitude, one we had talked about and hoped would never happen. But it did. Do I choose to keep Stephanie alive or believe the doctors and disconnect the breathing tube?

On February 3, 2007, Stephanie wasn't feeling well. She complained of a headache and was unable to eat much dinner. At 7:30, she was on her way to bed. This is highly unusual for her, the night owl, who usually is up until 11 p.m. or even later. I heard a loud BOOM as she went to bed and realized she had fallen down one flight of stairs, something she had never done before in her life. She hit her head on the wall, broke her right wrist, and had a deep cut on her left hand. After a few hours at the emergency room, the hospital released her with pending surgery for pins in her wrist. While at the ER, Stephanie was given a head CT, computer tomography, to confirm there was no bleeding on the brain.

Everything looked normal. That coming week she was laid up on pain medication due to the severe cut on her hand and her broken wrist. On Thursday, February 8, Stephanie had outpatient surgery to place pins in her wrist. She came home sleepy but feeling fine.

Friday, February 9, began as a normal day. She was feeling much better, moving around and talking about how frustrated she was because for a few weeks she wouldn't be able to work at the three south end middle schools in Seattle as a consultant. This concept drove her crazy. I reiterated that this was a blessing and she needed some rest, so take it. Anyone who knows Steph understands that resting is never an option when there is work to be done! Stephanie spent 15 years as a teacher and another 15 years as a principal. She could retire, but she was not ready. She began her own consulting company after she retired from Madison Middle School in 2001.

That evening I was busy working on my school district's budget. As part of the district committee, our job was to create scenarios that would cut two million dollars. Stephanie gladly offered to help. She was a great resource and was very coherent, creating alternative scenarios that even our Superintendent hadn't considered. I was having a difficult time keeping up with her and continually asked her to slow down and explain what she meant.

Suddenly, she complained of a headache and needed to use the restroom. Her face was the color of a ripe tomato, and she wanted a wet cloth for her head, saying she had never experienced a headache like this in her life. By the time I returned with the wet cloth, I could tell something was terribly wrong. She was in agonizing pain and was unable to talk. I helped her back to the couch and was about to get some aspirin for her head when a massive seizure began. All I could remember to do was to get her on her side and move all objects away. I managed to get her on the floor, propped up against the couch, but the seizure wouldn't stop. I didn't want to let go of her but had to in order to call 911. I had to go outside to the garage to access the switch to open the gate for the ambulances to get onto the property. By the time I returned to the house she was breathing but unresponsive. I was afraid she was going to die, and thoughts ran through my head at mach speed. What did I give her for dinner? Did I give her too many of her pain medications? What can I do now?

I was afraid she would choke because of the foam coming out of her mouth. She wouldn't respond. The 911 operator, bless her soul, kept me calm and had me keep talking with her and checking her pulse. The ambulances, yes, two, arrived within five minutes. They immediately moved me out of the way, rolled her over, and she actually began talking! Whew! I thought this was going to be a bad one, but she seemed to be coming around. As they loaded her into the ambulance, an emergency medical technician said to follow them to the ER as closely as I could. What was that about? She was talking and seemed OK. This type of response, my Pollyanna side, as others call it, came out often and was what kept me going.

On my way to the hospital, a mere five-minute drive, I called our dear friends Mike and Krissy told them to meet me at Whidbey General Hospital as soon as possible. I also called our friends Susan and Jenna in Seattle and told them what had happened. They were out the door and on the way to Whidbey Island within minutes. The hospital staff instructed Mike, Krissy, and me to stay in the waiting area while the doctors were doing tests on Stephanie. We had no idea what was going on, but we were all scared and anxious.

About twenty minutes later, we were ushered back into the ER. Steph's eyes were open, but she was not responding. The ER Doctor informed us that her CT showed a bleed in the brain, and the helicopter was on its way to take her to Harborview Medical Center in Seattle. I was in shock. How could this happen? I immediately told the doctor I was leaving so I could make the ferry and get there around the same time as the helicopter. His response was, "Don't leave her now; I am not sure she will make it until the transport arrives." This was the first time I knew how serious the situation was, but I just couldn't get my head to believe what I was hearing. All hell broke loose at that point. She started seizing again and her pupils were unresponsive. No fewer than ten people flooded around her. The doctor jumped on top of her placing a tube down her throat to keep her breathing. There were tubes attached and bells going off. The faces of the staff told the story. The situation was dire. I stood in shock watching as if it were an episode of TV's *Grey's Anatomy*. I wish it had been.

Luckily, our neighbors and good friends who both work at the hospital heard about the situation and arrived (small town, small hospital – I will forever love it). Jochen, a doctor, explained what was happening and showed me Steph's brain scan on the computer. There was clearly something wrong. A huge dark mass engulfed half of her brain. Finally, the helicopter arrived with four paramedics. I pleaded with the paramedics to ride in the helicopter, but they emphatically stated, "No!" They whipped Stephanie out of there before we could say anything. It was a surreal feeling watching that helicopter fly away not knowing if I would ever see her alive again.

After I called again, Susan and Jenna immediately turned around from the Whidbey Island-Mukilteo ferry terminal and headed back toward Seattle to Harborview. I also called Steph's sister, Dori, and her husband, John. They were on the way from their home in Gig Harbor. I returned home, called friends to meet at the house to take Ruby, our dog, and grabbed a few things, not knowing how long we would be gone. Mike, Krissy, and I headed for the ferry.

The trip to Harborview was excruciating--thoughts of Stephanie kept flashing through my brain. Did all of this really happen? Mike had the tough conversations with me during that drive, a conversation that no one else I knew would've been able to do. He let me know that my life as I knew it had changed. Best-case scenario, he said, she recovers and lives an ordinary life. Worst-case scenario, she is brain dead and I will have to make the decision to end her life. We talked frankly about the decisions I would have to make and that staying strong was the only way to get through the coming challenges. He assured me that no matter what happened, I would be all right. Life is tough, but the tough get through it. I knew I had to get my head ready for what was sure to be a long, frightening night. The conversation, although very hard, helped calm me down and realize that I could handle whatever I had to face. I would not be alone.

We arrived at Harborview around midnight, and I immediately rushed into see Stephanie while Mike and Krissy looked for a parking place. Susan, Jenna, Dori, and John were surrounding Stephanie, as she lay hooked to numerous tubes and on a ventilator. A neurosurgeon resident arrived and explained that her situation was extremely serious based on the CT scans from Whidbey. He told me that if she survived she was likely to be a vegetable and might never be able to communicate. Discussions Stephanie and I had regarding living and dying rammed into my head. We had both agreed that if we were responsible for each other, we would be strong enough to end each other's lives. Even though we had those conversations, I wanted to avoid the possibility. However, I couldn't avoid it because the doctors didn't know her and couldn't ever know for sure how her brain would function. I knew that removing equipment, declining elaborate brain tests, or refusing surgery would close the door to her life forever. I wanted to try to keep that door open.

The doctor wanted a decision--unplug the machine or attempt to keep her alive. He was very clear. If she lived through surgery, she could have massive disabilities, ranging from the inability to speak, walk, live in her house, serve a meal, take a shower, or interact with others ever again. Based on the results of the MRI, magnetic resonance imaging, the doctors at Harborview rated her 5.5 on a scale of 1 to 5... 6 is death. With all this information, what choice did I have? I knew they had never had a patient as strong-willed as Stephanie, and if anyone could make it, she could.

At that time, I asked the doctor, "Can you guarantee me she will be a vegetable?" His response was, "No, we don't know everything about the brain. I can't guarantee you anything." I looked at Susan, Jenna, Dori, and John for reassurance and then told the doctors emphatically, "Get her to surgery and do all you can to keep her alive, NOW!"

CHAPTER 2

◆ ◆ ◆

Bone Missing

While Stephanie was undergoing many more scans and tests, we retreated to the waiting room on the second floor of the ICU. We were in shock and wondered why they hadn't rushed her to surgery right away. Wasn't her aneurysm still bleeding? How long were they going to let it bleed before it stopped? How much more damage was the hemorrhage causing? These thoughts were on everyone's mind as we waited anxiously for any news to reach the waiting room. I had to get away from the chaos. Susan nodded and we stepped out into the hallway where it was quiet. I needed time to reflect, to understand the events of the evening.

During this time, the back elevator doors opened, and a patient emerged being wheeled from surgery to the ICU. As the entourage of hospital staff passed, Susan and I noticed that he had undergone brain surgery. He had tubes attached to his head, and a nurse aided his breathing. We also noticed large lettering written with a black sharpie pen on top of the dressing of his head that read in all caps, "BONE MISSING!" At first we thought we had misread the sign and were wondering, if it's missing, where was it, and why was it missing? Did someone take it? For some reason that sign stopped all the tears, and we began laughing hysterically. In hindsight I am glad I witnessed it, because that's exactly what we saw when Stephanie returned from her surgery hours later – all caps, "BONE MISSING!" Who gets to write that, I wonder?

Here's how things unfolded. About 3:00 a.m. a doctor named Nate Nare came up to discuss Stephanie's further test results. The results did not look good. One massive aneurysm had burst and was bleeding, but they also found a second aneurysm, which had not yet burst, but they were afraid that additional surgery could cause a major hemorrhage, which could kill her.

Their plan of attack was to do two surgeries. One surgery was required to clip the bleeding aneurysm. Once Stephanie was stable from that surgery, surgeons would return to clip the second aneurysm. It was a long shot, and Dr. Nare did not sugar coat his words. If she could survive the two surgeries, there was still no guarantee what her quality of life would be. For the remainder of the night and into the morning, we sat with Steph in the ICU, and I prepared myself for the very worst.

She was taken to surgery around 10:00 a.m. on February 10. We were told that this would be a very long day and not to expect any news until later in the afternoon. We had many family members and friends there with us throughout the day. We reflected on how Stephanie had touched all of our lives. While we were talking, it was very clear that all of us were wondering what was going on in surgery downstairs. I thought we were lucky that at least the doctors were giving her a chance by attempting the surgery. However, I couldn't help but wonder what she would be thinking if she were in my shoes. I envisioned her downstairs outside the operating room knocking on the windows wanting detailed updates as the surgery progressed. That is just who she is. Would I be able to fight for her as much as she would for anyone she loved?

At 3:00 in the afternoon, Dr. Nare came up to tell us things were proceeding and Stephanie was hanging in there. He didn't give us any other details except that the surgery would be a few more hours. We did not understand the hierarchy of neurosurgeons at Harborview at that point and thought Dr. Nare was her surgeon. Everybody was asking questions, and all I could think was, let him get back to the operating room. It wasn't until much later that we realized he had nothing to do with her surgery. That was left to the big guy, Dr. Laligam Sekhar, whom we had still not met. We continued to live in a state of emotional limbo, but our hopes were somewhat restored. She was still alive.

Seven o'clock in the evening came and went without a word from Dr. Nare. I needed to walk and get away from that waiting room. The waiting room had six other families all dealing with tragic situations like ours. Sometimes people communicate their pain and want to share the story about their loved ones. I didn't. I couldn't stand to see so many others in pain anxiously waiting as we were. Jenna and I decided to get a cup of coffee in the downstairs cafeteria. When Dr. Nare couldn't find me in the waiting room, he ran down to the cafeteria and approached us with a huge smile on his face. "They were able to stop the bleeding on the burst aneurysm and clip the second aneurysm with one surgery!" he exclaimed. That was great news for all of us! She not only made it through the surgery, but also would not need a second one! We ran back upstairs and waited for her to be pushed out of the double doors from surgery. When she finally came through that door, there were many of Stephanie's fans, seeing her head half shaved, tubes coming out, a nurse aiding her breathing and that God-forsaken sign, "BONE MISSING!"

◆ ◆ ◆

CHAPTER 3

ICU Psychosis

We had all survived the first twenty-four hours. As we set up camp on the second floor ICU waiting room, we all took turns sleeping and spending time with Stephanie. She was never alone. The nurses and doctors told us about the long recovery she would have ahead of her. This was the time we needed to get some rest, they said, because she had a one-on-one nurse. We heard what they were saying. Even though she was in a coma, I couldn't help think that maybe having loved ones nearby would give her extra strength. I nixed the idea to rest, and we continued to talk and be by her side twenty-four hours a day.

The brain surgery had caused massive swelling on the left side of her face with awful bruising. They had shaved the front half of her head leaving her long hair in the back matted with dried blood. She had five tubes draining the fluid from her brain, her "BONE MISSING!" sign, and a breathing tube. A sight for sore eyes! We began referring to her as our "girl with the mullet," I am not sure she would have appreciated the humor, but we needed something.

Many people were calling and wanting to visit. During Stephanie's time as a teacher and principal, she developed positive connections with students, parents, and teachers. She spent her time in those roles helping everyone be successful. She had supported them, now they wanted to be there for her, to know how she was doing, and to offer help. The last thing Stephanie would want was for anyone to see her in that condition. Stephanie's conversations and presentations with staff and parents had one point that was always at the top. She wanted everyone to understand that every child is a unique individual just like every adult. Success occurs only if all of us recognize that and respond to it in our daily interactions with kids. That also applies to interacting with adults.

While she was unable to make the decisions for herself, I would make them for her. I created a list of people who were free to visit and left that with the ICU nurses. Under no circumstances was anyone allowed in who was not on that list. Clearly that list was a reflection of what I believed Stephanie needed. I wasn't paying attention to adult individuals I didn't even know and hadn't seen my list. Those individuals, and there were lots of them, didn't know me, but they clearly had one thing in common. They wanted to see Stephanie themselves because they so loved her.

Where is my principal?
(A reflection from Bonnie Block, a former teacher and good friend.)

My friend Sherrill and I were interviewing at Aki Kurose for a job Stephanie had recommended us for: that's where I was when the principal asked if we had heard about Stephanie. We had not, so she filled us in on the little she knew. Fear rose in me when I heard the words, "…may not make it." I was too stunned for any questions. We went home, and I began making phone calls to determine where Stephanie was and what her condition was.

I don't remember when I decided to go to the hospital; I just knew that I had to go. I got lost driving, but eventually found the hospital and Stephanie's floor. A nurse told me how to find her room, so I began walking in the indicated direction. I wasn't looking at room numbers, just at the patients in the rooms. I passed a room where an older, bald man lay covered to the neck, apparently sleeping. It was hard to look at him because he was very swollen. I couldn't find Stephanie's room, so I returned to the desk to ask for help. The nurse asked who I was, and then walked me to the correct room. Immediately I felt sick. The bald man with the badly swollen face and the awful incisions was Stephanie, my principal, someone I admired, respected and liked beyond words. The nurse retreated, and I stood by Stephanie's bed talking quietly to her for several minutes. I was afraid to touch her. I was afraid she was

going to die. I was afraid I hadn't told her how important
she was to me. I was just afraid.

A woman came into the room and stopped short when
she saw me. I didn't have any idea who she was, but it was
clear by the look on her face that Stephanie was important
to her and I wasn't. I quickly held out my hand, smiled,
and told her who I was. She asked how I had gotten into
Steph's room, and she seemed quite upset when I told her
that a nurse had showed me the way. The visitor turned
out to be Paula, the person clearly in charge of protecting
Stephanie. We left the room and returned to the visitors'
area where Paula explained Stephanie's condition and
what was being done to save her. She was in an induced
coma, though I don't remember why. Paula told me about
the fall at home, about the seizure, and about what had
happened in the emergency room. It was a lot to take in all
at once. Other friends arrived, Susan and another person.
They did not seem as worried, probably because they had
known about things from the start. I stayed until I felt bet-
ter. Funny thing to say, isn't it?

The fight was just beginning. The doctors indicated
that Stephanie's biggest struggle would be to overcome
something called vasospasms that usually begin to occur
between days seven and fourteen. Vasospasms are caused
from the swelling of the brain after surgery when the veins
are not able to pump enough blood into the brain. They

shut down, and she could have a number of strokes and die. Five years ago, they had limited medications for this, but now they perform angioplasty to open up the vessels to the brain and allow the blood to flow. Each day they tested her blood flow to indicate the severity of the spasms. That was our number one concern, and we waited to see how severe Stephanie's would become. Another major concern was the extubation, the removal, of the breathing tube. I was so anxious to know the extent of the injury. I wondered if she could talk, recognize anyone, be coherent, or just lie there and be a vegetable. Sleeping in the ICU waiting room, I would dream that the tube was removed and she woke up saying, "What happened? Get me out of here!" I dreamed that her memory was intact and she talked as if there had been no damage to her brain. Did I make the right choice by keeping her alive? The anxiety was overwhelming.

The first week the doctors kept Stephanie in an induced coma to combat the swelling and keep her calm. This was the toughest time because we were awaiting the "awakening." I began communicating through the CaringBridge website to update people on Stephanie's progress. In essence, it was more of a support for me and allowed communication with friends and family that didn't require hours on the phone.

The following are my first week's journal entries and family and friend's emails.

CaringBridge Entry Thursday, February 15, 2008, 5:44 a.m.

Stephanie is currently under sedation for pain and on a breathing tube. When not as heavily sedated, she is able to open her eyes and look around. She responds to voices and touch. She absolutely hates her breathing tube and her left arm needs to be strapped down so she doesn't rip it out! (That's the Steph we know and love.) These are all great signs.

Email - Thursday, February 15, 2007 - 9:44

Many, many prayers going your way! Ruby says Hi and she misses both of you! If you need anything, Call Me! Thanks for letting me know about the site.

Angela Horton

CaringBridge Entry Friday, February 16, 2007, 9:05 a.m.

This morning Stephanie was responsive to touch and actually followed a command from the nurse. She squeezed her hand and put her thumb up. This is the first time she has been able to follow directions since the surgery, but we know Steph....she never has liked to follow directions, so this probably is a first.

Watching Stephanie for the first time follow a direction was very emotional for me. While she worked hard to get that thumb up in the air, tears rolled down my cheeks. It had been one week since the dreadful night and the first indication that she might really recover! It was all I needed to see and gave me the strength and reassurance that I had made the right decision.

Email-Friday, February 16, 2007, 5:07 p.m.

Stephanie

My thoughts are with you. You're irreplaceable, so even when life hands you such a difficult challenge, fight on! So many people value the good things you've done and we need you back.

Sincerely, Deanna Barrett

By Sunday, February 16, Stephanie's vasospasms were rated as severe, which meant if they didn't take action, she would have a stroke. Late that night the doctors performed an angioplasty, opening up the blood vessels and forcing more blood to the brain.

Email - Saturday, February 17, 2007 - 11:46 a.m.

Dear Stephanie,

You are always in our thoughts and prayers. Our Madison days always stand out and continue to shine because of your exemplary leadership. Our children need you.

Love, Lauren Divina

CaringBridge Entry Sunday, February 18, 2007, 4:58 p.m.

After the scan this afternoon, it has been decided to do another angiogram and possible angioplasty to help open up the vessels to her brain and increase the blood flow. An angiogram is an ex-ray test that uses a special dye and camera to take pictures of the blood flow in the artery. Angioplasty widens an obstructed blood vessel. This will be done tonight –

Email - Sunday, February 18, 2007 - 7:24 p.m.

Dear Stephanie and Paula,

I want you to know that I am praying for you every day. Stephanie, you are a fighter and have the strength to get through this. Michael and I send you our love and prayers.

All our love to you.

Julie and Michael Haskins

CaringBridge Entry Sunday, February 18, 2007, 9:50 p.m.

Stephi was back tonight! The angioplasty worked wonders and opened up the vessels allowing blood to flow to her brain. She was VERY responsive afterwards – she nodded her head in agreement to questions and shook her head when we told her she was going to have some more tests tonight – that wasn't part of her plan tonight ....we are sure she wanted to sleep after a rough day. We told her that many people were thinking about and loving her very much and she nodded her head and got a tear in her eye. She is very aware you are all out there. We are optimistic the angioplasty will decrease the spasms and help her heal.

Email - Sunday, February 18, 2007 - 10:50 p.m.

Dear Stephanie,

I'm thinking of you and sending good thoughts your way. You have been such a positive influence at Aki; we need you back. There's a whole school out there counting on your leadership. Come back to us soon.

Colette Blangy

Each day the doctors would do rounds at 6:00 a.m. They were easily mistaken for a flock of snow geese. The "flock of white" would rush into the room with Dr. Sekhar, the lead neurosurgeon at the front, flanked by a plethora of interns. He had an aura about him that expressed patience, kindness, and power. The nurses gave the updated report to Dr. Sekhar in a language that was incomprehensible to me. I was usually emotional and had a million questions. Dr. Sekhar would give me a quick smile, a squeeze on the shoulder, and his constant reply was, "She is going to be fine." I looked forward to those few precious minutes with him each day.

During the next week, Stephanie continued to be on the breathing tube and sedated. She developed pneumonia and was continually monitored for vasospasms. When she was awake she would immediately lift her hands and try to remove the breathing tube herself. At one point she got her left hand around the tube and would not let go! From that moment on, her hands were tied down. She would just stare into our eyes as if pleading with us to help her understand what happened.

Email - Monday, February 19, 2007 - 9:35 p.m.
Hi Stephanie and Paula,

I love this site. I am so addicted to it already. It keeps me up to date on the progress. We miss Paula lots, and hope to do half the job she would do at the WASL curriculum night tonight. All of our thoughts hope and prayers are with you. Remember caretakers and cheerleaders need to take care of your selves also. You are essential to the healing.

Jane Johnson

Email - Wednesday, February 21, 2007 - 11:59 a.m.
Hi Stephanie,

Neighbors Frankie and Jochen here. Paula has been giving us periodic updates and we are THRILLED to hear that your temperature has gone down. We're hoping that soon you will get that nasty tube out! And you will be able to talk again and tell everyone what's on your mind! That will be a cause for celebration for sure! We are keeping a watchful eye on your house and property. Every time I look over there I think about where you will put those goats. In addition, the llama, of course, to take care of the coyotes. Our thoughts are with you and Andy and Peter ask about your condition every day… Keep up the good fight Stephanie. We all need you to get better! And Paula, if you need anything when you come home (a hot meal, etc.) please don't hesitate to call over here!

Love ya,

Frankie, Jochen, Andy and Peter

Thursday, February 22, the team decided it was time to remove the breathing tube. The day we had been waiting for. It was a tough sight to see. Once the tube was removed, she was immediately put on oxygen and medication to help open up her lungs. She was still battling pneumonia, and breathing on her own was very difficult.

CaringBridge Entry Thursday, February 22, 2007, 9:39 p.m.

Today at 2:15 the medical personnel removed the intubation tube from Steph and she fought like a trooper. At this point, the tube is still out – she is exhausted, but her oxygen and carbon dioxide levels are still within the limit.

They are monitoring her closely and doing everything pos-
sible not to put the tube back in.

CaringBridge Entry Friday, February 23, 2007 10:41 a.m.

Stephanie made it through the night off the tube. They
had her on medication to help her breathe and have taken
her off of it this morning.

CaringBridge Entry Friday, February 23, 2007 7:07 p.m.

Stephanie did well off the medicine and should be able
to breathe on her own from here on out. She is still awake
and very unaware of what is going on or what happened
to her. We still don't know the extent of the injury. All of
her energy right now is spent on breathing. She looks good
– her bright sparkling eyes give us hope.

Email - Friday, February 23, 2007 - 1:42 p.m.

Hi Stephanie, Paula, and Susan,

Thanks for the updates. I keep hoping I will be able to visit soon.

Saw some of the golden apple awards last night and they were so inspiring because most of those recognized, acknowledged that they could only do what they do with support. It was so touching to hear one recipient thank all his favorite teachers from the past.

Stephanie, your life's work still pulses along in those you've touched, sustains, and makes us proud to know and love you. Keep trying. We believe in you. We are amazed at the progress you are making and continue to make.

Love, Kathy, Paul, Mary, and Helen Meyers

By Saturday, February 24, Stephanie was breathing with help from the oxygen mask. Her throat was raw from the tube, so any attempt at speaking sounded like Darth Vader. Nothing made sense. She was confused and didn't seem to recognize anyone but kept making gestures toward the door. She wanted out of that place. The doctors kept reassuring us and told us to be patient. Time would tell. I am not a very patient person by nature. Anytime the nurses weren't around, I would remove her mask and keep her talking even though her oxygen levels dropped. It was more important to me to hear one sliver of clarity. The lights on twenty-four hours a day, room temperature set to 54 degrees, and constant attention from the medical staff force people to lose their senses, especially the sense of time. Taking her mask off wasn't my fault. Blame ICU psychosis on that one.

On Monday, February 26, the ICU team had cleared her to move out of the ICU and into a program they called "step up." That floor was designed to focus on patients with traumatic brain injuries and had a ratio of two patients to each nurse. Prior to leaving the ICU, I was alone in the room with Steph when she woke up and said, "Hey, hey, hey!" I asked her if she knew who I was and her response was, "No, but no one's here. Let's go…NOW!" The nurse walked in moments later and her eyes showed she was clearly deflated. She lay back down and said, "Shit!" I knew at that moment, our Steph, so dearly loved was in there somewhere. I had made the right decision to keep her alive, and we were on our way to recovery. What I didn't know was how difficult that would be and how I wished I had taken the nurses' advice and got some rest during the time she spent in the ICU. For the next six weeks sleeping would be the last thing I did.

Email - Tuesday, February 27, 2007 - 1:10

Dear Steph,

They say that the basic character of an individual never changes.

I probably should "warn" the Harborview doctors about you. They have a strong, determined fighter on their hands. I'm reminded of us YEARS ago when we were staunch advocates for teachers' rights in the Everett School District. Harborview is an amazing place. Miracles happen here everyday. Dr. Sekhar is the best in the country at what he does. I'm thrilled and relieved that he was your surgeon. I'm pulling for you…and am willing to help however I can. I'm just downstairs from your room.

Hugs of strength,

Pamela Katims Steele ("Old" friend and current Harborview employee)

STEPHANIE'S BRAIN IMAGES

cerebral angiogram – left internal carotid artery – anterior – posterior view 2/11/2007

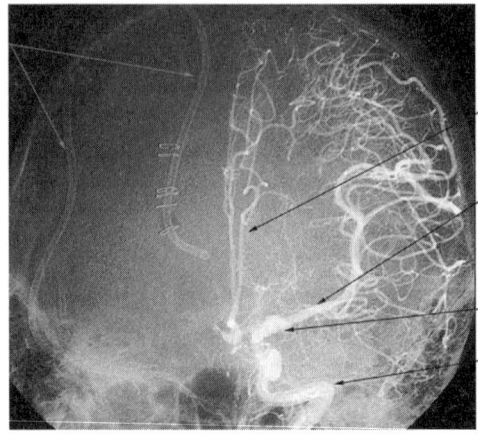

external ventricular drain (EVD)

left anterior cerebral artery

left middle cerebral artery (MCA)

aneurysm

internal carotid artery (ICA)

cerebral angiogram – left internal carotid artery – anterior – posterior view 11/25/2008

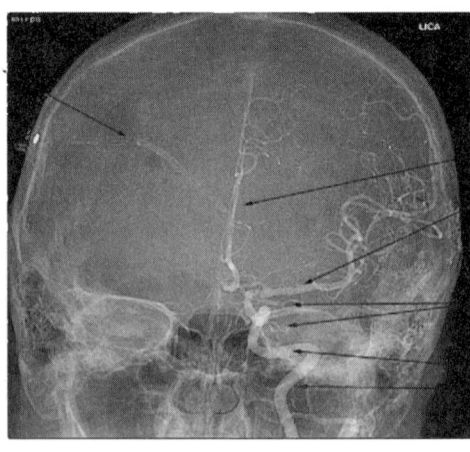

ventriculo-peritoneal shunt

middle cerebral artery

anterior cerebral artery

aneurysm clips

internal carotid artery (ICA)
• ICA cavernous portion
• ICA petrous portion

cerebral angiogram – left internal carotid artery – oblique view 11/25/2008

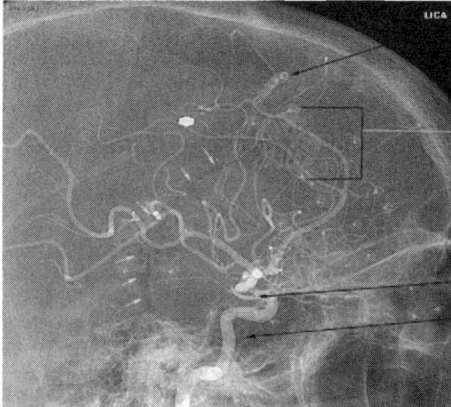

cranioplasty bone flap (outline in white arrows)

ventriculo-peritoneal shunt

titanium plate (for bone flap fixation)

anterior cerebral artery

aneurysm clip

internal carotid artery

clipping of an aneurysm

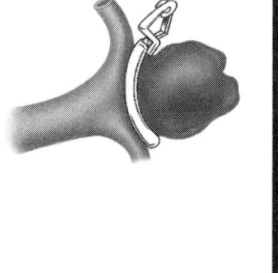

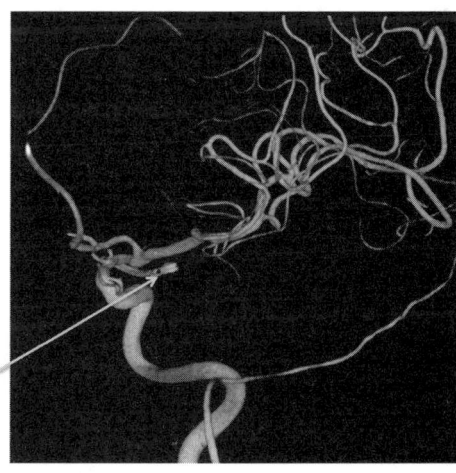

Stephanie's clipped aneurysm

CHAPTER 4

◆ ◆ ◆

Houdini Lives

The next month would try every ounce of patience I had. Even though she had moved out of the ICU, Stephanie was not out of the woods. The Neuro Specialty Unit was on the third floor at Harborview. It specialized in patients with traumatic brain injuries, a category Steph fit. She was still on oxygen and a feeding tube and was now in a room with another patient. She slept peacefully for the first two days.

Then she developed a horrendous fever of 104. The doctors were concerned that she had an infection in her spinal cord and that forced a regimen of lumbar punctures better known as "spinal taps." These are extremely painful. A large needle is placed into the spine between the vertebrae and spinal fluid is extracted for analysis. On Stephanie's first puncture, she used some choice words and hand gestures I had not seen for a while! Very appropriate for the situation, I might add. At least we knew the foul language center of her brain worked. They continued this procedure each day draining fluid to release the pressure in the brain and testing the fluid for infections. By the third puncture, they resolved to knock her out with medication. It was the only way they could complete the procedure.

Harborview is a teaching hospital so doctors were constantly on rotation for a limited number of days. Once a doctor became accustomed to Stephanie's personality and medication, the rotation changed. Regarding the amount of pain medication and the procedure that worked for her, there was little communication between the doctors. This caused great anxiety in Stephanie and her middle fingers got a work out.

By the end of the first week in her new room, she was talking much more. In fact, she talked non-stop. I felt that she was directing a staff meeting or attempting to hire a teacher. The tone of her voice and her nonverbal means of communication were the only hints one could use to determine meaning. She was now using real words strung together but made little or no sense. She ended each monologue with, "What do you think?" This caused immediate anxiety because she expected a response. My typical one was, "That sounds great."

Email - Tuesday, February 27, 2007 9:11 a.m.

Stephanie's transfer to another room, no matter what they call it, is great news. Does it, however, make her "escape" easier? When one gets an update so early in the morning, it is almost frightening to open it. I should have remembered that time has no meaning in the hospital, especially in ICU. Again, take care of yourselves. We miss you Paula and send positive thoughts to you.

Jane Johnson

Between lumbar punctures and the various activities they had planned for her during the day, I would flip through the TV channels looking for something other than soap operas to watch. Usually she paid no attention and could not focus on the screen. On March 5, I was flipping rather quickly when she told me "Go back… I like that one." *50 First Dates* happened to be her very favorite movie. She had seen it over twenty times. In the movie, Lucy has short-term memory loss and wakes up each morning forgetting the previous day. How ironic. I stopped on the channel, and she sat up in bed fully engaged. I wasn't sure how much she understood, but soon enough she said, "Oh….here comes the funny part!" She was right on. She knew that movie by heart, laughed at the appropriate times, and had the biggest smile on her face. I was feeling rather confident after the movie was over that if she could remember a movie then she definitely would know who I was. When I asked her, the response was, "No…and by the way, how much are you getting paid to do this job?" "Apparently not enough," was my only thought. However, this was the first coherent sentence she made, so my hopes lifted!

Email - Thursday, March 5, 2007 5:05

I'll keep my fingers crossed. I hope you (Paula) saw the Bob Woodruff story...it'll be a similar story for Stephanie I'm sure... the brain is so fascinating because it can rebound from such injuries. It is great she's verbal and I hope she gets better and better. My whole family wishes you as quick a recovery as possible. Know that if you need our help, we will be there. Your leadership at Madison has helped so many, but you still have work to do. Get well so, together we can all be better and continue on this journey with you.

Kathy Meyers

As she continued to gain strength, her resolve to leave the "hotel," as she called it, became her only goal. Because she was still missing a section of her skull she was required to wear a helmet anytime she was out of bed. She could take about six steps with assistance but was not allowed to walk by herself. Getting out of bed without help was forbidden. That is one command that never registered with Stephanie. She was restrained when she was in the room alone. This began with just two wrist restraints and a bed alarm. It didn't last long as she easily bit through one restraint and then untied the other to get loose. When the bed alarm went off, she was caught. Finally, she had wrist restraints, leg restraints, bed alarm, and a locked belly belt. That should do it they all thought. However, one morning I arrived early and found her lying on the side of the bed. During the night, she had managed to bite through both wrist restraints, unlock the side of the bed, and wiggle most of the way out from under the belly restraint. The sight was shocking. Diapers down to her knees, hospital gown up over her head, and her naked bruised body exposed. She took one look at me and said, "Could you help me out here?" I knew then we were in for trouble.

Each day Stephanie continued to regain her strength due to the physical therapy she received. The stronger she became physically, the more difficult it was to keep her contained and safe. She was still having trouble expressing herself, but it was very clear she was ready to leave. The doctors had scheduled to send her to rehabilitation full time, but the infection in her spinal column and the fact that her brain was not able to absorb the fluid was keeping her on the specialty floor. Until they could get those two issues resolved, she was stuck. Susan and I took Stephanie for walks each day. We each supported one side by holding onto her arm. Her left side remained weak and without support she would teeter and tip over. One day she was able to walk from her room out into the hallway. As we walked past the elevators, she turned, gave us a smile, and bolted! It took all our strength to hold her back. She couldn't articulate verbally, but we knew that she recognized the escape route.

We left that night informing the nurses to "Beware… she has seen the elevators!" At approximately 4:00 a.m. I received a call from the head nurse. During the night, Stephanie had bitten through both wrist restraints, untied her leg restraints, and managed to squeeze under the locked belly restraint. She then headed for the elevators! She made it about ten steps before a nurse could respond to the bed alarm. As they hollered, "Stephanie, stop!" She turned, lost her balance, and fell back against the wall just outside the doors to the third floor. Of course she did not stop before her escape to put on her helmet. She ended up putting a two-foot hole in the wall that would remain there throughout her stay and was quite the conversation piece. They rushed her down for a CAT scan, and luckily, all scans were negative. She landed on her shoulder and the back of her head. Her response when I arrived was, "It's not my fault." After this escape, she was given a single room directly outside the nurses' station where every movement could be monitored. This wouldn't be the last time Stephanie would receive such specialized treatment.

Another reflection from Bonnie Block.

At first, I was amazed that Steph could actually speak and move around. However, it didn't take long to see that whatever she was saying wasn't making any sense to anyone else in the room. She talked about work and people I did not know. It was altogether sad and funny to listen to Steph's "original" words and expressions as she tried to make herself understood. She asked many questions of me and of Barb, but she had no ability to process our responses. Her manners were evident when someone came into her room. She would welcome everyone with something like, "Hello. It's so good to see you." However, the empty look in her eyes told the true story — she had no idea who the person was. Nurses and cleaning staff got the same greeting as friends and family. I found that empty look to be both innocent and terrifying. Over and over, I wondered if Stephanie would ever be once again the Stephanie who had turned Madison into a school to be proud of.

I guess that's all except for one thing. The communication made available through the CaringBridge was truly a lifeline to Stephanie's progress. Paula will probably never know the importance of the entries she wrote. I can't speak for anyone else, but I know how I felt every time I found a new entry. I rejoiced at the good news and suffered with the bad. But through it all was a slow progress that gave me hope for Stephanie's recovery. Living through this experience with Stephanie in the small way that I did changed me. I live more in the moment and I express my feelings to people I care for more easily.

While strapped down at night Stephanie decided to re-move the IV's by using her teeth. She knew enough not to complete this task during the day as I was there and more nurses were present. Each night out came her IV! Soon the doctors decided that a PIC line was required in order for her to receive a heavier dose of antibiotics for the infec-tion, not to mention that most of her veins had collapsed. This would require placing a line into an artery close to her heart. The doctors were skeptical that she might try to remove that as well, so they decided to stitch it into place. That should do it they thought. Nope it lasted all of thirty minutes. They had restrained her wrists so she used her mouth. Out came the PIC line! I returned to witness blood all over her and the bed. She was beginning to become a handful and my twelve-hour days were turn-ing into seventeen or eighteen hours. I was afraid they would not accept her full time into rehab if she continued to act this way, and I did not want to see her in a nursing home facility. I could only imagine what would happen -- LADY IN BLUE HELMET LOOSE! The thought was overwhelming.

Within two days they had put in a new PIC line fas-tened with something similar to duct tape, impossible to remove even for Stephanie. As they continued with the lumbar punctures, it became evident that her body was not able to absorb the brain fluid. A shunt would need to be inserted in her brain to drain the excess fluid to her abdomen. The surgery couldn't occur while she had an infection in her spinal fluid. I knew we were not leaving that room for some time.

While she recovered from the infection she was more determined than ever to leave. I knew I had to be there with her during the day or she would be confined to the restraints. I couldn't imagine how scared she must have felt alone. She did not understand where she was, she did not recognize her loved ones, she did not understand what had happened or why we were still staying in the "hotel." This fear caused her to scream incessantly if family members weren't at her side.

Soon our days became a routine. She would wake up and get ready for the day with help from Occupational Therapy and Physical Therapy. All of this was completed by 10:00 a.m. and that left me the rest of the day to keep her occupied.

As soon as Stephanie started to cry and complain about needing to leave, we would use the huge orange bags that Harborview provided for patients to pack their belongings upon discharge. We would spend at least an hour clearing the entire room. The articles included her personal belongings, syringes, towels, bedpans, toothpaste, pillows and anything else she could find. When this was completed and our Harborview cart was full of at least 10 bags, I would tell her she had to take a nap before the car arrived. While she took a nap, I would unpack everything and wait for the whole scenario to play out again. That process occurred about four times a day. She never remembered that she had already packed. As soon as she woke up the first thing out of her mouth was, "Are we ready to go?" My immediate response was, "Well we have to pack first." The process would begin again. *50 First Dates*...no wonder it was her favorite movie. She was living it.

Soon the entire situation took its toll on both my body and emotions. I could not face one more day of packing, lumbar punctures, and constantly trying to understand what Stephanie was saying. The most difficult aspect for me was getting glimmers each day that she recognized me and knew I was important, but they were fleeting. Is this how it would be if she ever made it home? Would she ever know my name? Was I just another nurse to her? I began to lose hope that I would ever have my partner back. I began to feel very alone and afraid.

By the grace of God, there were nurses on that floor that were fabulous and very patient. One nurse in particular, Ethel House, RN, or Queenie, as everyone called her, nicknamed Stephanie "Whippersnapper." She understood the impact of brain injuries and was the most amazing human being. She loved Stephanie and always took time to listen and try to understand what she was saying.

One day as we were packing for the second time, I began to cry. I was exhausted and couldn't do it one more time. Queenie told me to take a break and the nurses would not restrain Stephanie, but look after her. Forty-five minutes later, I rounded the corner to the nurses' station and was utterly shocked! There she was helmet on backwards, sitting in a swivel chair, busy as ever! The nurses had set up a workstation for Stephanie complete with an unplugged fax machine, computer, and phone. She was talking on the phone, typing on the computer, and seemed to be in Heaven. When I asked her what she was doing her reply was, "I can't talk to you right now, I'm kinda busy." One nurse would say, "Stephanie, you have a call." When she would pick up the phone and no one was there she would curse the person out for hanging up and go right back to her work on the computer. The problem arose when an actual phone would ring and she attempted to answer it, which happened more than once. She beat the nurses to the phone more than one time. This usually ended in her hanging up saying the person was "nuts" on the other end of the line. We now had a new routine. At least two hours a day Stephanie had "work" to do at the nurses' station.

Finally, March 19, the infection in her spinal column had cleared and it was time to put in the shunt. I begged the nurses to shave her entire head during the surgery because of my feeble attempt with Wal-Mart mustache clippers. Her surgery went well and she returned with a clean-shaven head. This was a vast improvement over the initial mullet. Her incisions were reopened and she now had a huge lump on the right side of her head. Within two days it was clear the shunt was working as her spinal fluid began draining into her abdomen. We were finally getting out of this unit and on our way to the fourth floor and rehab.

Prior to getting into rehab at Harborview, one had to qualify. Stephanie was required to answer an array of questions. If they weren't correct, then her destination would be a nursing home. When Stephanie was asked a question she didn't know the answer to, she let it be known that there could be multiple answers depending on how someone looked at it. Her explanation and answers were amazing but incorrect. When asked what animal grazes in the grass? Steph said that it could be any animal. The lion could be chewing on a meal in the grass, and a giraffe could be leaning through grass to eat leaves, and a chicken could be hiding, and the horse could be getting ready for a race. Each question had four answers. Stephanie came up with an explanation as to how each of the four answers could be correct.

Stephanie was with them for an hour and they asked her one question after another. I could sense that she was very nervous and knew this meeting was important. Based on Stephanie's answers, the creativity of them, and the number answered correctly, she made it into rehab. One step closer to home.

CHAPTER 5

◆ ◆ ◆

Please Return to the Nurses' Station, Now!

Would she be back? **(A reflection from Barbara Greenlee, former teacher and good friend.)**

Her language was very weird. She greeted us with "formal" phrases. I realized that this had been learned. It was something along the lines of "thank you for coming to see me." I realized immediately that she had no idea who we were. Paula introduced us with a "you remember Barb and Bonnie" phrase to cover the situation and the awkwardness. She smoothly lied and started to speak in the language I call Steph aphasia. The structure was there—sentence syntax, inflection, pauses at the right points when put together. I think. But the nouns, verbs, adjectives, and adverbs made no sense. Mostly she said real words, but they made no sense when put together. She was trying so hard to be understood, but I don't think at this point that she knew what she said made no sense. She would ask a question and we would fake an answer or tell her we didn't understand or best, didn't know.

When she was talking during this time, it was impossible to understand anything she said. However, what she was saying was very important to her. She was extremely earnest in whatever it was she was saying. I found that to listen to her I needed to not listen to the words, just to the sense or heart of what she was saying. I may have been putting my interpretation onto her words, but it seemed that she was working through various thoughts about her work and family. She was processing some disagreements and problems she had. Sometimes she would come to a conclusion. I could tell from the tone of her words and her body language. She would ask something that required my agreement. If I asked her an open answer question (Do you think that's right?), she often answered clearly "The important thing is love and friends. The other things aren't important now." She would then relax for a bit and then start in on another "problem." She had to get her "work" done.

Later visits showed many changes. Steph got more memory and mobility each day. She couldn't read any words at all. She seemed to be about 18 months old cognitively, but had many adult concerns. She wanted to do the "right thing." She was concerned about time and her schedule. She could not tell time yet, so she asked what time it was and how long until her next appointment. If I told her 10 minutes, she didn't understand. I some-

times told her I would give her a warning, and sometimes showed her on the clock face when things were due to happen. (It's 10:15, when it gets to 10:30 you have to go to physical therapy—pointing to times).

As time passed, it seemed that Steph was going through all the stages in cognitive learning. She could negotiate like a 2-year-old who didn't want a nap or a 9-year-old who thought a playground rule was unfair. She was uninhibited about her privacy like a 3-year-old, and as shy and private as an 11-year-old girl. Each time I saw her there was a new person. It was hard to wait until she revealed how "old" she was when I got there. Treating her like last week was not all right. Neither was anticipating her development. I found that the best thing was to let her talk, ask her about herself, and describe how much she'd learned. She would then reveal her new development level. One week she would walk around the floor and look in every door and then not recognize where she was. The next week she could lead me to speech therapy. She would tell me to get her a "purple kite" when she was thirsty, and then could ask for cranberry juice. Where had the woman who could save teaching and schools gone? Would she ever be back?

I had known Stephanie for seven years and wondered where this drive came from. How did she continue to survive the initial aneurysm, major surgery, the ICU, and the weeks in the neuro unit? Her nurses began telling me they had rarely seen a patient like Stephanie and that the tough ones, patients who were so difficult to handle, were the patients who made the most progress. That gave me hope. Stephanie couldn't recognize her surroundings, couldn't articulate her needs, but knew enough to want to leave. Do all people have that, or was she unique? I thought back to all I knew of her and the many stories she told me of her past. Then, only then, did I realize that giving up had never been an option.

She spent a total of thirteen days in rehabilitation. At a pre-meeting it was stated she would be in rehab for one month. After a week in rehab they wanted her to go home as much as I did. Their mistake was made on day one. She was placed in a room away from the nurses' station and with a roommate. I had a gut feeling that the room arrangement wouldn't last long. She was very confused with her new surroundings and couldn't understand where she was and why she wasn't at home. With the freedom of not being in restraints she enjoyed visiting patients daily. Only a curtain separated Stephanie from her roommate, whose name happened to be Nanette. This reminded Stephanie of the play, *No No Nanette* and she constantly pulled the curtain back and stated with energy and enthusiasm, *No No Nanette!* to the utter surprise of her roommate. I was sure we were going to be kicked out, but instead they immediately reassigned her to a private room outside the nurses' station again with an absolutely beautiful view of Elliot Bay. This room came equipped with a camera and a wrist monitor that set off an alarm each time she passed the doors. "PLEASE RETURN TO THE NURSES STATION, NOW!" Too bad, she didn't understand what it said!

Rehab was frustrating for Stephanie and me. Our doctors repeatedly reminded us that the first eighteen months were crucial for the brain's recovery. The brain's progress slows down significantly after that window of opportunity. I knew we had no time to waste. We had to use each moment to regain and rebuild what had been lost. I knew as an educator that we had to focus on the essentials of reading, writing, speaking, and comprehension. Stephanie needed a daily schedule to be large and visual, and that is the thing she focused on throughout the day. Every afternoon we would create the schedule for the next day. We kept the previous day's schedule for her review.

Daily Therapy Schedule

8:00 Breakfast

8:15 Brush teeth

8:30 Wash Face

8:45 Change Clothes

9:00 Not assigned

9:15-9:45 Speech Therapy

10:00-10:15 Break

10:30-11:00 Occupational Therapy

11:00-12:30 Break/Lunch

1:00 Speech

1:15 Speech

1:45 Physical Therapy

2:00 Physical Therapy

2:15 Physical Therapy

2:30 Occupational Therapy

2:45 Occupational Therapy

3:00 Occupational Therapy

Hospitals are using the same rehabilitation methods for all patients. Brain-injured patients receive the same curriculum. Why isn't it individualized? Isn't that what we have learned works best for children? Why should brain-injured patients be any different? In order to evaluate the program and the needs of all the patients, these questions needed to be answered.

Occupational therapy was ridiculous. The questions they asked: Will ice cream melt in the freezer? Do plants need sunlight to grow? Can you borrow books from a library? Can a fly walk on the ceiling? This frustrated Stephanie because she wanted to trick them to get out of there but didn't know the answers. "Does pork come from sheep?" Stephanie's response was, "No, not physically, but then farmers might have them on their farm and because the sheep did well, the people could also have pork." She didn't know. Who created this craziness?

Here are more examples from Occupational Therapy.

Task 1: Completion of Categories: List one or more things that belong.

1. apple, cherry, banana _____*lime, lemon*_____

2. roast beef, chicken, pork_____

3. ankle, foot, neck_____

4. shoe, hat, dress_____

Task 2: Identification of Object Described: Write the word for each.

1. Babies like to play with these. _____*toys*_____

2. It is found on a car. _____

3. People drive these. _____

4. We sleep in it. _____

Task 3: Phrase Completion for Final Nouns: Finish blank to finish each phrase.

1. A pair of_____*shoes*_____

2. A loaf of _____

3. A piece of_____

4. A bottle of _____

Another requirement of occupational therapy was getting ready each morning. This meant Stephanie showering, getting dressed, eating breakfast, and brushing her teeth. Early on we gave her support with these tasks. One morning, Dori and I helped Stephanie in the shower when she decided I needed a shower too. The showerhead came off its hook before I had time to do anything and was turned on me! I had no other choice but to hold her up, close my eyes, and get soaked. Apparently my earlier shower didn't count for Steph. She laughed and gave her usual response, "It isn't my fault." I began to think these charades were her fault and she knew exactly what she was doing.

Speech therapy posed the most difficult challenge for Stephanie because she did not have many words in her brain that made sense. She would fill her mouth with three or four pieces of gum before each session so if she didn't make sense they might think it was because of the gum, not her words. I don't think she fooled them with that trick!

The therapist showed Stephanie pictures of a man's tie, his suit, a giraffe, and a cow. Really? Is that what is important, knowing the word for tie? Will she ever use it? Our time was limited, and I was becoming as frustrated as Stephanie. Why should we worry about labeling a tie and suit when she didn't even know my name, her pets' names, and labels of common household items? My knowledge of student learning kicked in. I became very involved in her rehab and I'm sure a major pain in the ass.

Stephanie should be identifying and naming things and people from home. Now didn't that make sense! Her speech therapist agreed that was a good idea. She began to realize that it was hard to name items while at the same time she was extremely frustrated that she couldn't identify her surroundings. She would look at the picture of our dog, but not ever be able to identify her by name. She would say, "Hey….I like that."

One goal for Stephanie's discharge included cooking. The expectation was that she go to the grocery store and create a meal on ten dollars. Stephanie's meal included French toast and bacon. I had never seen her eat or cook French toast! Luckily, my best friend David and I were there as witnesses to this extraordinary event. As we arrived at the grocery store, I realized what a ridiculous situation the rehab facility had created. Here was a woman in a helmet, having eaten hospital food for nearly two months, and being set free in a grocery store. David and I followed Stephanie as she attempted to buy the food in order to make her French toast and bacon…laughing all the way because it didn't take long for Stephanie to find the peanut M & M's and any other sweet she had been missing the past months. Each time the therapist asked her to read the signs to find what was on her list; Stephanie just returned to the snack aisle and filled her basket with sweets. That exercise felt to me like checking something off the rehab list and was not beneficial for the patient. Watching from afar, I wondered who created that idiotic task. Upon leaving the grocery store, David and I had many sweets to snack on and a lot of laughs in the process. What a ridiculous task for anyone to complete, but what great laughs for my best friend and me!

She was required to cook the meal. Very emphatically she declared, "I do not like French toast." She settled for scrambled eggs and burned bacon. I don't think she passed that particular rehabilitation goal. I wouldn't dare to think of letting her cook at home or be loose in the grocery store at that point.

At the time of discharge Stephanie's doctors identified several goals:

Stephanie must be able to:
- Safely walk indoors 150 feet.
- Climb up and down stairs using only a handrail.
- Accomplish daily personal hygiene with little or no help.
- Perform household activities, including cooking, laundry, cleaning, and personal finances with little help.

During this time she referred to me as, "The one who helps me get home." I began to hope that she would recognize her surroundings and also me. I had waited months for her to "know" and "recognize" me. I finally realized a single sentence or word would not accomplish this. It was the combination of words, small gestures, and her constant need to be home that gave me this hope. Even though she couldn't articulate our relationship, I thought she knew who we were.

CHAPTER 6

◆ ◆ ◆

Klockerbogs

Steph was more than ready to come home when the doctor set her release date to April 5, my birthday. I was overcome with both excitement and fear. I wanted to be home, to be with the animals, and look at Mt. Baker on a sunny day. I was tired of spending hours at Harborview and feeling "lost." I was also afraid to take her home. Could I take care of her? What if she didn't recognize the house or animals? What if she didn't get any better? Could I really do this? Nobody understood how scared I was. I had already taken five months off work and knew I only had the summer to help her recover. I felt very alone and fearful of the future. I decided to put those fears aside and let the real adventure begin. I had no idea what an adventure it would turn out to be!

Steph seemed to relax with each mile as we began our trek up I-5. As soon as we got off the ferry at Clinton and started driving up Whidbey Island, she was fast asleep, awakening only as I drove down our long driveway. The real questions were about to be answered. Would she recognize anything? She got out of the car without a word and proceeded straight to her couch, grabbed the TIVO remote, and began to search for her favorite shows. In the hospital, we worked endlessly to teach her to push the "nurse button," funny she could never accomplish that task, but was a master at that TIVO remote. I knew then she knew not only her house, but also me.

I let her rest for a couple of days, and then the real work began. Dori, Stephanie's sister, is a special education teacher in Gig Harbor. One of her specialties over the course of her career was working with students who suffered from brain injuries. This knowledge was valuable as we created an intense rehab regimen. It takes courage to do the right thing despite the fear. I had to utilize the time. The schedule encouraged Stephanie to read, write, talk, listen, and do physical activities. I also wanted her out in the community daily working on communication skills.

The following list was posted on the refrigerator with times included. She would often go look at that list to find out what was coming next!

Daily Activities
1. Hand Exercises
2. Practice Picture Identifications Flash Cards
3. Medicine AM and PM
4. Distance Walking

5. Writing in Journal
6. Blood Pressure Monitoring
7. Helping cook Breakfast, Lunch, Dinner
8. Reading magazine or newspaper and retelling what was read.
9. Watching a TV program and retelling the story line.

Additional Activities

a. Trips to the store – once or twice a week
b. Coffee shop
c. Appointments when needed
d. Speech Therapist Meeting two sessions each week
e. Visiting friends
f. Clean the house
g. Physical Therapist – once a week
h. Working outside in the garden

Life was incredibly busy at home. My favorite time of day was Stephanie's naptime, which meant going outside for me. Her constant need for naps allowed me, with monitor close by, to weed places that had never before seen daylight! The busier I kept her in the morning, the longer nap she would take. It seemed a little selfish, but trying to interpret her speech was exhausting. She was like a wind-up doll with no off button.

The handwritten journals became an overall important part of her rehabilitation. I knew as an educator that her injury had affected not only her expressive language but also her receptive abilities. I was hoping that a combination of journal writing and practice with speaking, listening, and reading activities would help to maximize the eighteen-month recovery period. I also knew I had to go back to teaching in the fall, so my goal for her was to be independent by September. After Stephanie wrote in the journal, she would give it to me to read and comment. Most of the time I had no idea what she was referring to, but I gave her positive reinforcement nonetheless. Inwardly I chuckled at her made-up words and wondered how much better they would get.

Her beginning journal entries were difficult to understand. That was also true of her spoken language.

Home Rehab Journal - April 10, 2007

Red feel talked – real conversation – talked with tala from school saw over feed becks spense – talked johnin the sumner on Friday for weekend – also talked about fsso on Saturday.

This entry was a good example of her early language ability. Constantly I was in a state of panic attempting to decipher the meaning from her words. She would ask for her "klockerbogs" but was unable to gesture what she meant. Was it her shorts? Did she mean eyeglasses? What about leg sheets? I finally figured that one consistently meant sweat pants. Whew! On one occasion around dusk as we drove into the driveway, Stephanie shouted, "Look, there's a bee!" She is deathly allergic to bees. I slammed on the brakes, made her get out the car, and frantically began batting away inside the car looking for the bee. She was confused and asked what I was doing. She had been looking at two beautiful deer grazing down by the trees and flowers not far from our house. Bee? Deer? She said the words were close enough!

Welcome to my life! Her speaking was as good as her writing. Imagine that.

Home Rehab Journal - April 11, 2007

Mayor and ages – then came to visit bringing her hersband to lose with – fix bathroom-

Chores – beat on a fire in place – fire house – fed the cats and spent then – made coffee-clean flier.

Live on a listening we went to strategy with antrol pink poll – we went to talk about a system – to divine how we use. Use writing to put in dubey-meant for it to use.

I remember this journal entry very well. I slept in past six that morning only to wake up to hear commotion upstairs. Immediately I panicked. Did she put her helmet on before she walked upstairs? Did she try to make coffee? I sprinted upstairs with my heart in my mouth afraid of what

I would see. There she was sitting on the stool in front of the fireplace, helmet on backwards, with a beautiful fire burning. When she saw me she said, "I was hot." I realized it was time to increase her list of chores to include feeding the cats, unloading the dishwasher, and putting her own clothes away. Many surprises came out of this – soymilk with pots and pans, spoons with the onions, and when she didn't know where it went, the refrigerator was her best bet! Two years later, we were still finding things in strange places.

Coupeville is a wonderful, small community and a great place to recover from an injury of this magnitude. The patience of others and their willingness to assist Stephanie as she struggled to communicate was amazing. On our daily excursions, she was responsible for writing checks, ordering coffee or lunch, picking up her medications and grocery shopping. Often it took over ten minutes to get a simple task completed, but no one complained. I am sure she was quite the sight. Away from Harborview there aren't many people walking around with a head full of scars encased in a shiny blue helmet.

Home Rehab Journal - April 13, 2007

Role on stuff field machine. Donna went off to acknowledge some real estate. We went to SDD demonstrated – got my glasses skicked, got Paula' windshield faced, parking strip – went to grocery to buy for groceries.

Home Rehab Journal - April 14, 2007

Steph and Dori sat and pay peal paid peavey pulled around agreements and – Steph learned a lot about disecese. Dori, Steph, and Paula went on jove jepp and had coffee. We all postad for all which was quick and delicious.

Home Rehab Journal - April 19, 2007

We went on a traveling trip thing – we went to absence days – all said my arts were ok – I have incris in art and rare – just a month but should who be able to heck it off – it felt good. We were in society. We took a riverteria pass with no sudcak for riece, then we went to an Olympia part for dega typers and then to Sophia – who said that was her mother had been hought by that but she was theme with it – it was ok and isn't not satisfactory.

During our "traveling trip thing" on this particular day, Stephanie was trying to tell me something. I informed her that a word didn't make sense. She told me that I had a limited vocabulary and that the word was actually a word that made perfect sense! The word was "speekle." Anyone heard that one before? It really could have been my limited vocabulary.

As we continued throughout the summer with our arduous rehab schedule, her language began to recover and her physical abilities increased. By the end of July, she was driving by herself, and by early September, she was working daily on her computer. She was able to care for herself. Our goals had been met. I could return to work full time knowing she had the ability to take care of herself.

I wonder what it must have been like for her as I sit and reflect on Stephanie's recovery. How did she feel? What did she remember? Here is a person who had a very successful career as a teacher and principal and is now afraid if she doesn't do everything she's asked to do she will be sent to a nursing home. She would get emotional but rarely complained or showed frustration at her disability, even when she struggled to be understood. She has taught me that giving up is never an option. I feel privileged to be a part of her life.

I believe we need to understand Stephanie in order to know what to do for brain-injured patients. Her voice helps us understand the struggle and the amount of perseverance it takes to recover. Sharing her writing and reflections are the essences of this story. Her voice is the power.

Stephanie's Story

◆ ◆ ◆

CHAPTER 7

Trapped

My memories of the ICU are nonexistent. I did go back to visit the nurses on one of my trips to see Dr. Sekhar, and I remember nothing about them or the place that I stayed. Everything was unfamiliar. It is a strange feeling to be in a place where your life was hanging by a thread and to have no recollection whatsoever.

During my stay in the neuro specialty floor, I remember very little of any activities that occurred during the day. I don't remember hitting the wall, trying to escape, or working at the nurses' station. I also don't remember any of the lumbar punctures or shunt surgery, which I guess is a good thing.

One vivid memory I have is the first time I saw my reflection in the mirror. I remember looking down at the water in the sink. I looked slowly up to see myself in the mirror. It was freaky. I didn't look like myself at all. My head was naked with short hair all over. My scar was surrounded by fat tissue. My eyes looked like they were barely there as the side of the skin around them came down. It was the first time I realized how bad I looked and how much I had been through.

People were there during the day that I recognized and made me feel safe. Maybe that is why I have little memory of this time. I trusted the nurses who worked with me during the day. I was comfortable with them for the most part. Then when they left, the night terrors started. The medical staff thinks patients won't remember, but we do. Brain-injured patients who can't communicate their needs and are unable to use the TV remote or use the call button for help have limited options. While I understand now that being restrained was for my own safety, I wished there was something they could do to help communicate that to me. I hope that people in medicine can look at this situation and figure out an alternative way to keep patients safe.

The memories during the nighttime are very strong. They are actually nightmares and revolve around being tied down with no one willing to help me. I thought they were trying to kill me. I realized in retrospect these memories occurred at night when I was alone. I couldn't move. I could not comprehend what was happening to me. Where was everyone? Why would no one help me? Why were they trying to hurt me?

The following entry is from my home rehab journal I wrote on October 23, 2007, eight months after the aneurysm, obviously a painful memory.

Home Rehab Journal - October 23, 2007

I started working on the ropes. I didn't understand why I had to be tied up and not allowed to move off the bed. I could not talk people into letting me not be tied with white cord. Some of them would not be as strict as others but they all used the rope. They bother me. One night I tried very hard to get them off but covered them so people will leave me alone. I had to be careful. I would loosen the rope on one hand and then the other. It took almost two hours. The night nurse answered that she was angry. I said I am a good person who does not like being tied up. It is hard to do nothing. I can't stand it. I think it was horrible. Someone I didn't know told me to stay in the room. I tried to be funny and use a joke so she couldn't tie me up. She said the only way is if people stay here with me. I needed someone to help me get away. Hospitals need better ways.

I still have nightmares about night nurses and night-time. I cry every time I talk about it. I felt like the night-time nurses, in particular, were playing with me – entertaining themselves at my expense. My memory was of them standing in the hallway looking into my room and laughing. They frightened me as I thought they were plotting to hurt me during the night. Another behavior I remembered was the nurses taking my TV remote and changing the channels or turning it off when I wanted to watch something. They also tied me down too tightly so I could not move my hands, scratch my face, or roll over to lie on my side. They wouldn't come to untie me when I had to go to the bathroom, I felt petrified that something could happen and I could die. There was no one to help me at night. I was trapped.

There were many nights that the nurses ended up calling Paula to return to the hospital to calm me down. One particular night she had left around 5:00 p.m. and was driving to Anacortes, 90 miles away, to spend the night with her good friend Kelly. She had just arrived when she received a phone call from the night staff that said I was out of control and she needed to return. She spent a total of 20 minutes with Kelly before leaving to return to the hospital. I didn't learn about this until much later, but now I am thinking some of those night nurses can't even do their jobs!

I spent all my time at night trying to escape. Wondered where I could go and then I made a plan. I thought I just could get on a bus. Eventually the bus driver would notice I wasn't getting off and take me to the police station where they could deal with the situation. I didn't think about the fact that I had on an adult diaper and carried no money.

I still want to face the people who are responsible for supervising night nurses. I would like to explain how I felt and why. We need to work together to find a better solution to this problem. I recognize now that I was a very difficult patient because of the damage to my brain. I am certain that if someone ever tells them about my opinion they will say that it is me not them. Of course, I have an injured brain, so surely I am not able to tell the truth.

The truth is I am not the only one.

Email - Wednesday, March 13, 2007

Hello Stephanie,

My name is Gary Paine. I am a friend of Jordan Gussin. I have been following the updates on Caring-Bridge and understand what you are going through. I went through (about 8 years ago) aneurysm, brain surgeries, coma for 3 days, ICU, tubes, summer in hospitals, the whole nine yards. I read your journal and it brought back memories of things like all sorts of tubes coming out of me, not wanting to be there, frustration with not being able to communicate. I too, ripped some tubes out and tried to escape in the middle of the night. I got about three feet before I collapsed on the floor, with a little voice going. "What are you doing? You don't know how to walk anymore!" Anyway, my story ends happily. I was 50 when I had the stroke. Eight years later, everything has come back except balance. I still tip over easily and I am very uncoordinated and walk with a cane. (I miss skiing, racquetball, and volleyball). But that is a small price to pay for being alive and being surrounded by family and friends. I go into kindergartens and sing songs with children, and the response I get makes being alive worthwhile. I wouldn't go through it again for anything, but I do have an appreciation for all the love and wonderful people there are in the world.

When it became apparent I was getting close to leaving rehabilitation, I was scared because Paula was going home for three days to clean and prepare the house for my arrival. She tried to explain to me that no one had lived in the house for the past two months. Things needed to be done. I kept negotiating with Paula and didn't understand why I couldn't come and just sit on the couch. I promised I wouldn't get in the way. Paula's going home frightened me. It was my first memory of her, and I was afraid of her leaving. Susan was with me for the three days and my attempts with negotiations didn't work with her either. I didn't believe I'd ever get home.

Two months at Harborview and my most vivid memories are of nighttime. They are still very strong with me today. I wonder if they will ever go away.

CHAPTER 8

◆ ◆ ◆

Playing in the Sandbox

Being at home was wonderful because I was out of the hospital. I was not tied down. I could walk around whenever I wanted. The rule was I had to wear my helmet at all times, and I could not go down the stairs unless I had someone with me. That was easy to follow compared to the demands they used in the hospital.

Home was peaceful, and all I wanted was sleep, rest, and to talk to Paula, whose name I couldn't remember. In fact, Paula wrote her name on a little strip of paper and taped it on my watch. That way I could look at my watch to remind me of her name. Prior to this, I had called her Tom, Pam, Pat, and Hey. My favorite one was Hey. With her name on my watch, I now had a chance for the future.

The peace didn't last long. I had two days of rest before the work began. Paula told me I needed to follow the daily schedule posted on the refrigerator. I struggled to remember to go to the refrigerator and felt I didn't need to follow a schedule. I knew what to do in my house, but I wouldn't be able to stay at home if I didn't follow the schedule. I felt Paula had complete control over me. She was like a teacher, and I was a first-grade student. She controlled what I ate, what I did, and what pills I needed to take. The only thing I controlled was the TIVO. I realized then I wasn't free.

One important task was relearning words I needed in order to communicate. Paula took photographs of family and friends, my clothing, and some of my things. Each photo was placed on an index card with the label on the back. Suit and tie were not on the top of the list. Harborview could take a lesson from Paula. My job was to say the name of the photo without looking at the back of the card. This felt funny to me. I didn't believe I needed to work on those words. I knew what they were. I knew my socks went in my shoes. I knew where my shorts went. Why was it important to know the name? I was scheduled to do this activity multiple times throughout the day. It caused great anxiety because I knew I would get it wrong. I would describe the picture and hope Paula wouldn't ask me to name it. I tried to distract her and cheat. How would she know leg sheets meant sweatpants? Government injustices meant taxes? Scissors meant my eyeglasses? Humdingers are hummingbirds? I still can't get that one right! Why was she doing this to me? I guess at the time I didn't recognize the importance of learning the words.

We did many activities in the community. I got excited when we left the house because I thought I didn't have any assigned work. There was more work than I anticipated. One time we went grocery shopping, and my task was to write the check. The problem was I didn't understand months, numbers, or words. That wasn't easier than being at home. The checkout line was getting longer and everyone was looking at me. I didn't like that, but I did like riding in the car.

Part of my daily routine was reading. I picked up a magazine every morning and selected one or two lines to read to Paula. I would try very hard to find a meaning I could share with her. I remember trying to read. I had told Paula I knew enough and I didn't need to practice anymore. She told me that I needed to understand what I was reading. I knew that I couldn't understand the magazine but thought she didn't know because I kept that a secret. I would read several magazines each week and newspapers before the aneurysm. Now I struggled to understand what happened and even who the people were.

The one that struck me the most is the *Newsweek* feature called "Perspectives," which came once a week. It quoted seven to ten well-known people. There were one-liners with a short explanation. I picked the easiest one at the beginning of the week. I would read the quote and the information. I looked for something I recognized: a title, a state, or a person. I didn't understand any of it. I could barely do one or two. I could fake it the first couple of days, but by the end of the week I was out of options. I had a hunch Paula knew I couldn't read or understand it by the look on her face.

Another daily task was twenty minutes of writing in my journal. I found this easy because I could use big letters to fill the space and didn't have to use correct words. I could just write, and it wasn't graded. Paula would ask me to read her the journals, and I couldn't. She would read them aloud and tell me I did a good job. The rules were the house had to be quiet, no TV or radio, and no talking. I was supposed to focus on my writing, but all I wanted to do was talk. I felt like Paula had to remind me of this continuously throughout this exercise. Remember where I was headed if I didn't follow the rules? Paula won.

I switched from talking about myself in third person to first person after only ten days of journaling. That was amazing because it was a tremendous change in my brain. For the first time I could see me. If people cannot see themselves, they cannot grow. Getting to that point is a huge door being opened.

Home Rehab Journal - Wednesday, April 18, 2007

They are watching a play. One that Stephanie and Paula sell apart. That is a great flya. It is relative nice. Paula meant suicide and stayed and talked with them. The impressionment was pure. Mary, Aimee and Theresa joined the conference. I got help with names because I'm not nameless yet - & touching them-speaks-but is not there for the same-the teacher for the spark know is not near-but we had a visit of him-the two split on the muddy occur-is compination of visits and trees-some combos-fantasy-by my brother includes my brother and dad whom are dead-prim who leads my strength who does in fact.

On Friday, April 20, while at Harborview for an all day doctor's appointment Paula and I had three hours to kill. It was very important to me that I communicate with all the people who were supporting me for the past two-and-half months. Paula suggested I post something to the Caring-Bridge site. I thought this would be easy. The following entry took me three hours to type. I made many mistakes and had to rewrite it many, many, many times. My final version still wasn't perfect.

Home Rehab Journal - Friday, April 20, 2007

Hello Everyone

This is Stephanie here on the computer and I wanted to take a minute to thank you for your support. This has been amazing and I have been amazed at what it takes. I have been supposed at my home trying to pull the neceissities together. The communities' support of my effort has helped me make progress day by day. Thank you…..thank you. Hope to see all of you when summer roles around.

Love, Stephanie

It was wonderful to have people respond directly to me.

Email - Friday, April 20, 2007 11:58 a.m.
Hi Stephanie,

I read your thank you note today and it made me cry... with relief I might add, just to know that you have demonstrated your great courage and come so far in the healing process in a relatively short time (I'm sure that depends on who's arm the watch is on!) I know that the blue sky and sunshine will help regrow and resodder those synapse. I look forward to visiting you on the island this summer. It will provide a good reason to relax on this end as well.

Always my best!
Bill Mason

Email - Friday, April 20, 2007 3:15 p.m.
Stephanie,

I am soooo pumped to read your very own words. It gave me goose bumps; I could just about hear your voice. I am so very happy for your recovery and I can't wait to see you!!!! It sounds like you are doing great. When Mac and I came to visit you in the hospital, I knew you would be back to your old self and even better before I knew it. Congrats! Paula we haven't met but you are truly amazing!! Can't wait to hear more.

Jasmine Riach

Email -Tuesday, April 24, 2007 6:11 p.m.

Hi Stephanie and Paula,

So fun to have a first person entry from Stephanie and glad to hear everything continues to go well and improve. We love you both sooooo much and look forward to seeing you soon. Hugs and kisses.

Kris and Riley

I also went to outpatient speech twice a week. My injury was so severe that my speech therapist, Susan, coined my aphasia as "global," meaning I was unable to understand what was being said and unable to communicate effectively my own thoughts. I could see things, but I couldn't speak about them. I felt like since I was writing in my journal I was making good progress. I wasn't reading what I had written or was feeling like. I had to do more to understand what I was thinking. After watching me recover in August, Susan regained her hope in the ability for patients with global aphasia to communicate again.

I was beginning to read what I wrote. I indicated that I was checking the sentences to some degree. I found in one sentence that I wanted to say "neater" but used "meter." I caught it and said something about it. That was the first time in over a month of writing that I noticed and looked for mistakes. My journal still had problems despite this. I talked about what people are doing and I wrote, "Pam's going hiking." It was actually Paula. I think people who don't have brain problems do not understand or pay attention to how effective your brain operates under an unconscious umbrella. You are busy, talkative, expressive, all coming out of your voice or what you have written to others, sometimes to yourself. At that level, you don't pull back, become quiet, and see the umbrella far above you. That is where everything comes from.

Home Rehab Journal –Monday, May 14, 2007, continues

I read the stuff from yesterday and hope to have – I wish everything looked meter –I mean neater – the book is on my thigh –I just got of talking for Dori. We had a dinner at lunchtime yesterday with Bev – neither. She nor her daughter liked it. I had to wear my protective cap. I tried to act good about it – She – Paula – didn't like all the wish feed – or white feed – I waited until they had a good one – the one you put in squares that was good – I think they were solving this just so people's need for food to have a small choice of typical breakfast was given out. I just remembered high muffin. Dori will be here this Friday and we are going to work on the deeds we need for may time – Also we need to work on a plan – to give away – Pam's going hiking with Kelly to hiking on Saturday. Names I want to remember: Bev, Paula, Dori, Kelly, Patrick, Addy, Susan, Jenna, June, Barb, & Georgette.

I also wrote about my protective cap. It is not a cap. It is a medical helmet required if you have a hole in your skull. Readers might ask why I am mentioning this. It's simple. Two years after the aneurysm when I was writing this, I was going to use the word cap. I looked at it and knew it was the wrong word. Then after about five minutes of trying to think of the right word, suddenly it came into my head. That umbrella that I mentioned earlier took care of it.

I attended a field trip to Deception Pass Park at the end of May with the first graders from Crescent Harbor Elementary. They were very excited and happy about doing a two-and-a- half mile guided hike. They identified certain trees, different kinds of vegetation, created and labeled pictures of animals and plant life. I had been home almost two months and had no idea how much I would connect with these students. I really was a first grader.

Home Rehab Journal –Thursday, May 29, 2008

A friend from the school agreed to drive me down to the field trip activity and I had to wear my protective cap. When I worked as a teacher and principal, we tried to make sure students wore appropriate dressing to protect them. At this time of year, shortly after almost dying in the hospital, I had an entire head shaved. I felt weird in an odd way. I knew that I was getting better each day when I did little tasks, and it was made total when I saw those six-and seven-year-olds try to do their learning activities. They were individuals, and it showed. One child couldn't remember trees, another couldn't spell the word to describe their sights, and yet others couldn't remember to look up high. As children experience like this, they learn about themselves and more things they need to understand and learn in order to grow and learn more effectively. When I watched them, I realized that they were my peers. Some things with my brain worked sometimes, and other things didn't work at all. It isn't like noticing what is not working, announcing it, and from then on expecting it won't be a problem or mistake going forward. The children on this field trip might have to be alerted about areas that need more development. Telling them about it, showing it, giving them practice on it, is one small step where many more steps in lots of areas and experience are taken so that eventually they know and understand.

They helped me realize that I had a long way to go. When you realize that every student in our country goes through this process every day, it is stunning. That process is what students have to do to grow and develop. It is adjusted to the students as individuals so that the support given to each child is what each one needs. Schools that manage the support for the individuality of each child result in to wonderful progress and success. Schools that don't do as well put students in groups and treat them in various groups regardless of the individual needs. I sat on a log on that rainy May Day in 2007 and watched the students walk by. On that day I knew that I decided I wanted to hear how each student was doing. I know that I realized that adults who go through severe injury to their brains and lived through it need to be treated as individuals. Just like children, every patient is unique and an individual. Rehab needs to help them improve and work back to where they were before the brain injury and related damages.

During this early recovery period my favorite time of day was the moment I opened my eyes in the morning, not quite fully awake, but peaceful. Maybe it's because my brain wasn't awake yet. I think it is probably true that from children to adults we never emphasized the notion that we would be stronger if, when we woke up, we simply stopped for a few minutes. We would think about our dreams, think about the room we slept in, think about the safety of being in that bed, and feel calm. Then, think about the day ahead. What will you need to do? Who will help you? Whom can you learn from?

This is how I felt:

Home Rehab Journal -February 2008

Each morning when I wake up there are just a few minutes before I come totally awake and I felt normal.

It is my bed and I slept well in it. I am warm and I feel peaceful. I look at the walls. They are white and crisp. My favorite large picture is framed on the wall. It is a picture by Georgia O'Keefe of a bunch of white clouds in the sky. It is like you are looking out of a plane at all the clouds and as if you were flying in a real plane it gives you the same feeling…that you could walk on those small clouds and jump from one to another. You know that they couldn't hold you up, but it seems like they could. It is a painting that reinforces how I feel now about things I look at and that seem like I could do something real with them.

I began to realize as I continued to make progress the impact this injury could have on the rest of my life. I didn't want to embarrass myself, have people not listen to me, or not understand what I tried to say. I wanted to fix it before it came out of my mouth. I would think of the word quietly so no one could hear it. That was safer for me and no one could tell me I am wrong. Talking with people continues to be great deal of work.

Would I always struggle to recall words? Would I be able to drive? Would I return to work? What would life be for me in the future? Thoughts like those, and many more, were constant and often terrifying.

◆ ◆ ◆

CHAPTER 9

One Block at a Time

Highlight of the summer: no more helmet. On June 22, 2007, I got my bone back! I was very tired of wearing the helmet but also nervous about having the surgery. My hair had grown back and I knew I would end up with another large scar and a funny looking haircut. I spent three days back at Harborview but this time avoided being tied down and could even use the TV remote. There was much pain involved in this procedure, but I was helmet-free. I often wore a soft, fleece cap on my head to avoid the stares people would give me with a half-shaved head and some nasty stitches. The hair had grown back enough within a month and I was ready for action.

CaringBridge Entry June 25, 2007

Stephanie successfully had her own bone (complete with titanium mesh) replaced on Friday, June 22. NO MORE HELMET! Of course, now we will have to wait like all the others in the long ferry lines.....no more pref-

erential loading. The doctor let me know they used a little Elmer's and some paint glue to make sure her bone was intact! She is now the proud owner of a "reverse mullet" and lots of stitches! A little early, but a great Halloween get up. We will work on the hairdo as it grows – what a treat to worry only about…HAIR! Can't wait!

Each day after the surgery things seemed to get better. The swelling was going down so when I got up to brush my teeth the stranger in the mirror was actually me. Living without the helmet was fabulous! Even though I had huge scars on my head and a big lump where the shunt was placed, I didn't care at all. It is almost as if my vanity disappeared. It didn't matter because it meant that I was alive.

Comprehending continued to be a struggle for me. Restaurants were especially difficult because of the noise, and I couldn't read the menu. I really had difficulty tracking conversations with more than one person. Interacting with people made me anxious, and I became exhausted.

The most amazing part of recovery was I couldn't see the difference between who I am now and who I used to be. You can't imagine you will move forward because you are trying to go backwards. There are many blocks in the way, and if you can't see them, how can you know what to do to take it down one block at a time. My journal entries in July showed the improvements in my language one block at a time. I was taking down those blocks.

Home Rehab Journal – July 7, 2007

Paula and I are up early and setting up things that need to be done this next – It will help me getting stuff that shows to feel like I feel better on my life – Paula is having fun & so am I to get things in done –including things to buy.

Home Rehab Journal – July 12, 2007

I get tired of writing my thoughts but keep trying to –Don't know why I'll make this work bothers me – If I could do this each day it would be better –I am slooping more & better – so this would influence it. Got a message that Barbara Green wanted to connect – I should probably green that – Did a loss of mess in my office area –better place that there was – and how it gets better.

Home Rehab Journal – July 13, 2007

Paula is great to work with. We got coffee & make sure all things made it to our house & make sure that we have lots of coffee & time to spend –We enjoy our way and look kindly to others.

I really wanted to start driving again by August. The doctors told me that I would need to be cleared by the state in order to be legal. We found out that was not true! It was a trick to make sure I stayed off the road. I was determined. I asked her every day if I could drive, and her answer was, "Not yet." I think she was afraid but I knew I was ready.

CaringBridge Entry August 2007

One sunny day in August 2007, we were on our way to town to get a decaf soy latte when Stephanie decided she would like to drive to the end of the road. I was nervous and wished I had controls on the passenger side of the car! She zoomed up the driveway, went to the corner, and stopped. Then she took a left went down to another stop sign. Once again, she stopped but then turned out onto the major highway. At that second stop, I thought she would stop and let me drive. Not to happen....she finally felt some sense of control over her life and took off down to town. This drive lasted for about thirty minutes as we toured through the town and down to the Port Townsend ferry dock before heading home the back way. She did great and had a new sense of confidence about her recovery. It is this moment when I felt she would be independent enough to make it once I went back to work in 3 weeks. Looking back through the recovery process after coming home, it is difficult to believe the struggles she endured to end up where she is today. It is as if nothing happened, sometimes a word is lost, a confused memory, but couldn't that be attributed to growing older and not a massive aneurysm? She is an amazing human being who has continued to push herself to the limit, not stopping until she feels "like her old self." Her old self is back, but a new sense has made her appreciate what life has to offer and her ability to see beauty in all things makes those who are fortunate enough to spend time with her, see it too.

I had done it! Driving was like riding a bike....just get back on and away you go. This gave me great independence and allowed me the freedom I didn't know I would ever feel again.

Our last event of the summer was fast approaching. My birthday was just around the corner, September 4, 2007. I have never looked forward to a birthday more than this one. I was alive! We were going to celebrate! That celebration would not just reflect the day of my birth but also celebrate the people who helped me survive. There was much to be thankful and happy about.

The party took place on August 25, 2007. Even though it was a Saturday in August and usually would be sunny, this particular day was cloudy but not raining. We brought in lots of great things for people to enjoy. We had hamburgers, steaks, fish, chicken, salads, rolls, and drinks. The property has five acres, so the families who brought children were able to let them play out in the acreage and participate in outdoor games.

I was anxious because I knew that I didn't talk nearly as well as when I was working as an educational consultant, a principal, and a teacher. Some people I didn't know well prior to the aneurysm had the chance to know me during my recovery. They could see how much I had improved over the summer. They only knew me by what I was like after the aneurysm. Even though I would have problems with nouns and sentences, I knew they wouldn't be very concerned. I felt very nervous about the people who had known me before the aneurysm. I knew they would notice me missing nouns, not making sense with each sentence, and with any questions I asked.

I used my birthday as an excuse to bring everyone together. That gave me the chance to thank them for the things each of them had done to help me improve. People want to extend to help, but they don't want to be given lots of clapping for it. I understand that especially now. That's how I worked with children, parents, and teachers. When we give support to a child or an adult, it is most important that the attention rest on the receiver. All of those wonderful people I knew saw me as the receiver and focused on me.

Birthday Messages August 25, 2007

Happy Birthday to one of the most miraculous people I know. The definition of "miraculous" and "accomplishment" has changed over the past thirty years I have known you. But, your beauty and warmth have remained a constant. Kudos to you my friend. You amaze me.

Hugs.

Pamela Katims-Steele

Happy Birthday Stephanie! I don't think I have ever been to a birthday party that made me happier than this one! Watching you recover is one of the most wonderful gifts I received. Much love,

Your speech therapist,

Susan Walker

Stephanie,

Sometimes I lose perspective on my life and think I need to fix, improve, repair, and redo. You remind me that my life is a gift… given to me everyday… each day… repeatedly. I am so GRATEFUL!

All my love and support.

Jenna Brown

It was a perfect way to end the summer. Now it is time for me to give attention and support to them so our friendships grow deeper. We had reached our goal. I had made enough progress to take care of myself, and Paula could return to work knowing all of the hard work had paid off! We had made it.

Final CaringBridge Journal Entry
Tuesday, August 16, 2007

Stephanie is doing great and passed her 6-month exam with the neurosurgeon with flying colors (she interviewed him for 25 minutes…shocked him senseless). He said,

"See you next August." He gave her the go ahead to drive on the island – yikes. Little does he know, we've already attacked that one.

He was amazed at her progress and indicated again to her that she is a MIRACLE. Steph again thanked him for keeping her alive and his response was amazing. He indicated that removing her aneurysms kept her alive, but did not give her life –it is her friends and family that helped her stay the course and have a reason to live – thank you all for that.

We wouldn't have our Steph if it wasn't for your support. Thank you and much love to all… Paula

CHAPTER 10

◆ ◆ ◆

The Hero

Laligam N. Sekhar, M.D., is the primary reason I have written this book. He is a brilliant neurosurgeon and the one who gave me a chance to live. Equally important, Dr. Sekhar balances his technical expertise with soul, heart, warmth, and compassion, qualities he extends to each of his patients. He models behavior we would like to see in all doctors.

Paula and I went to visit him in August of 2007 for a review and a CAT scan. We brought him vegetables from our garden. He asked me the names of the vegetables with a gentle smile on his face. I could describe the vegetables and their use but I couldn't come up with their names.

A question I could never answer while in the hospital was what kind of work I did. This meeting was the first time I could answer him. I was a teacher, a principal, and an educational consultant.

Our next visit was in November of 2008 to review the angiogram results. The results indicated that the repair remained successful. He shared with us how different I was in talking now from when I saw him in August of 2007. He recognized my growth. He let me know it, and he made me feel wonderful.

What I want to work on the rest of my life on this earth is supporting medical leaders like Dr. Sekhar to successfully communicate to people about brain injuries. I want people to be informed. It is amazing how in just the past ten years and particularly the last five years, the significant progress that has been made.

We returned in February of 2009 to interview Dr. Sekhar for this book. He also invited me to speak at a brain conference on aneurysms. The following are five excerpts from that interview with Dr. Sekhar and my comments at the conference.

Personal Interview with Dr. Sekhar
Harborview Medical Center
February 28, 2009

I think many health care professionals do not realize how well the survivors do over time. If you take your own case, the nurses asked why we are bothering with this patient. She is in bad shape, and she has not improved for so many days. I said you know that her brain doesn't look that bad. She is a young person. Let us persist with the full three weeks of treatment and see what she does. Guess what? At the end of two and half weeks, you started to turn dramatically for the better. We have had a few other patients like this. What happens to the nurses in intensive care units, they are very good people and they are very good about taking care of ICU patients, but they get burned-out syndrome. They feel sometimes that doctors are keeping patients artificially alive. The nurses have no frame of reference. The frame of reference I have is I see the patients when they come in. I see the patients in ICU. I see them in the outpatient clinic. Then I see you like this just now. Just this one patient has given me enough confidence and happiness to work hard to help the next 100 patients that are referred to me. But then nurses don't know that, because they are not seeing the patient longitudely. So that is an important thing to convey.

Senator Joseph Biden, who had a ruptured aneurysm and was treated in Washington, he did well. He also had another unruptured aneurysm which was treated. And here is now - the Vice President of the United States. Whether you are for him or against him doesn't matter. But the fact is he has reached a very high position. Right? However, he doesn't say a word about what happened to him. Why? He feels people will say, "Oh, he has had brain surgery, therefore he is a cripple." People will think that. No one wants to say anything about it. Right? This is the reason.

I think being physicians and being teachers probably come to nearly the top in terms of occupations. When you are a teacher, people may not give you enough thanks, but every time you see that student... Being a teacher has been compared to being a ladder, somebody said a ladder. Does anyone thank a ladder? No. But how many people climbed up that ladder to go to somewhere very important? Right? So, these are probably the top two occupations in any society. But, I feel blessed to be able to do what I am doing.

I also think further education can help these patients to manage their health better. I think that is where people can make a difference. By that I mean patients, organizations, and a book like yours. Not research into the condition, but what I find lacking personally, is support services for the families. You are very fortunate to have a circle of educated, reasonable people that support you. I have patients that don't have that.

One thing I remember about you all the time you were always surrounded by friends. In addition to your dear friend, there were always seven to eight people in the room, and they were laughing, they were joking, and we would laugh and joke. But always people there.

Stephanie's Presentation
March 10, 2009
2009 Mini-Medical School Graduation Night

Dr. Sekhar: *(Dr. Sekhar presents Stephanie to the audience)* I have with me today two patients, and one of them is Stephanie Haskins. If you can, come up for a minute. Stephanie was a former middle school principal. She came to us with a very bad ruptured aneurysm. She was in a coma for two and a half weeks in the intensive care unit. The nurses gave up on Stephanie. We just are going to treat her, and let's see what happens after three weeks. Miraculously she started waking up. She had surgery to clip the aneurysm. And now Stephanie is back. Stephanie Haskins. *(Applause)*

Stephanie: Thank you, thank you very much. I am so proud to be here tonight with my hero. *(Applause)* There is a team of people that support me; three of them are here tonight in the front row, my sister, my best friend, and my other best friend. All the other people who supported me want to hear how this went tonight. So, I am really glad to share with you and say…

When I was a principal, and when I was a teacher, when I worked as a consultant with schools in Seattle to try to do all the right things for kids and parents, you never thought of it happening to you. I didn't think of this happening to me. I thought they would say to me, okay let's get going. So on February 7, I had a phone conversation with them to talk about this really positive time going on at Aki Kurose Middle School in south Seattle. We were really excited, and yet by Saturday, he saved my life. I didn't talk to him for was it three weeks, four weeks, before I could even …

Dr. Sekhar: I talked to you. *(Laughter)*

Stephanie: That is why all my people, I mean well over a hundred people, they're friends I know and teachers I worked with, who came to see me. They wanted to hear about what Dr. Sekhar was saying and what he was doing. So I am sort of passionate now after a year and a half to two years working on this every day. I was challenged by people. I have to say this, I used to challenge them. I used to be a principal and I used to be their supervisor, and I hired them as teachers. I used to teach kids. And they all helped me.

Now, I would like to share that with anyone who goes through what you go through as you try to recover. Rehabilitate. But the most important thing I think I want to have you understand is I have the rest of my life, which we think will be a long time because I am working so hard every day. I have friends in schools that call me and still say, "Stephanie, you sound really good. It is time to go back to school." But, you know what? I am devoted to you and anyone who has gone through this. I want to do what I can to make it one that you survive and that people and all of us know about it, so you don't go through the one I went through. *(Applause)*

One last thing, Joe Biden, the vice president of the United States of America, had a brain aneurysm. He doesn't talk about it. I am going to write him a letter and going to see him, because there are people both famous and ordinary whom I care about. We need to all start talking about it because this is important work. And I think they want to hear me and talk to me, because, after all, I have Dr. Sekhar, the hero. *(Applause)*

Dr. Sekhar: Thank you so much Stephanie. You truly are a miracle. *(Applause)*

At the time of this lecture, we were all joyful and felt this battle had been won. It had been a little over two years and that night signified the end. I had made a full recovery except for those damn nouns!

In our wildest dreams nothing could have prepared us for what was coming. Battle number two was just around the corner.

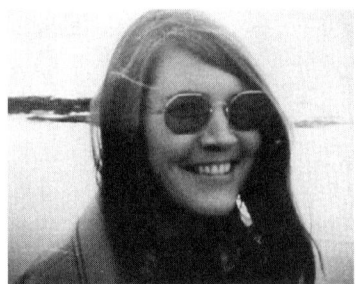

First year teaching 1970's...
style says it all!

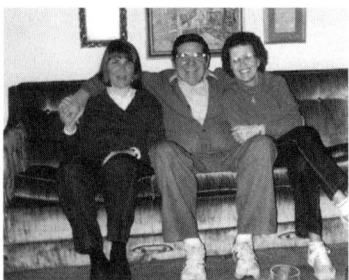

Mom and Dad taking a break from
their many selling schemes. I learned
a lot from them.

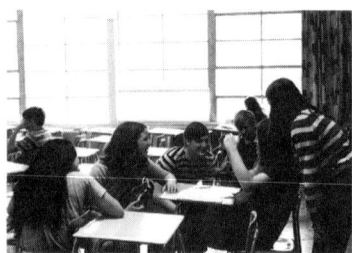

What was I explaining to my 9th
grade English class that kept them so
entertained? I can't remember.

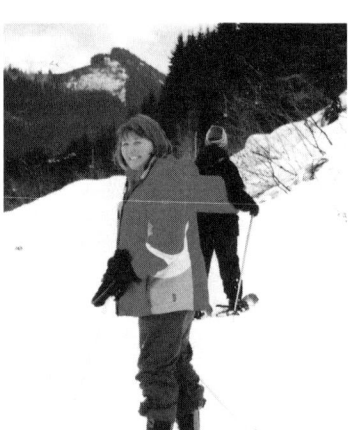

Snowshoeing on Snoqualmie Pass

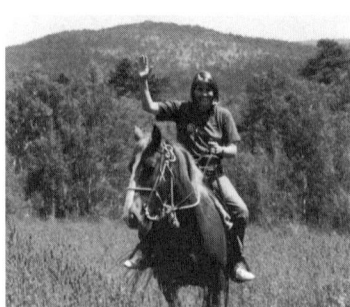

Horseback riding in Estes Park,
Colorado

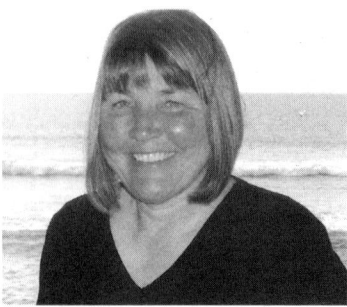

Maui 2004 pre aneurysm

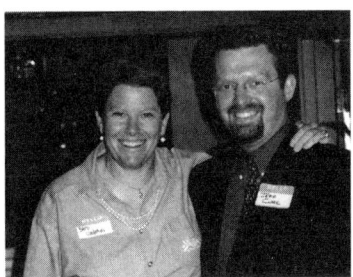

Barb Vadakin and Jeff Clark from Madison Middle School in Seattle. Both are great people who I was able to support and they in turn supported me throughout the aneurysm. Jeff is currently a principal at Denny Middle School in Seattle and Barb is enjoying many trips to Hawaii.

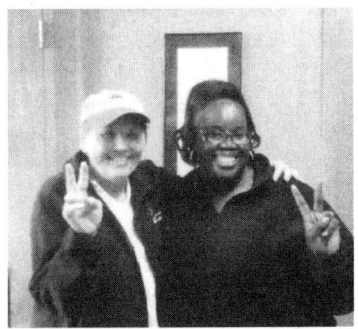

Mia Parker Williams, another great supporter and current principal at Aki Kurose Middle School in Seattle.

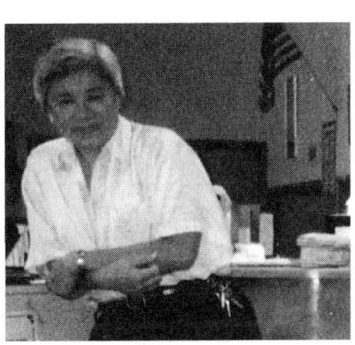

Bi Hoa Caldwell, colleague, friend and previous principal at Aki Kurose Middle School.

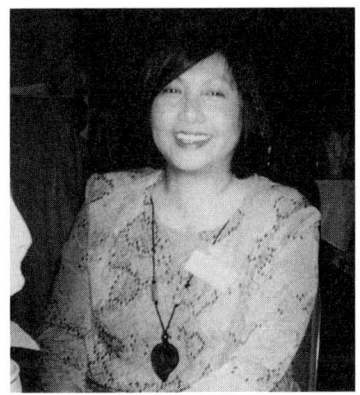

Lauren Divina – wonderful counselor at Madison Middle School.

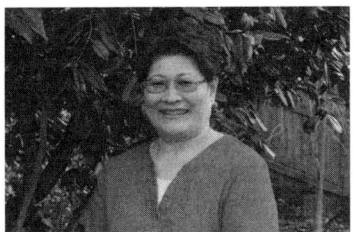

Georgette Kinoshita worked as the financial assistant at Madison Middle School and eventually the budget manager at my consulting company. A great friend and supporter.

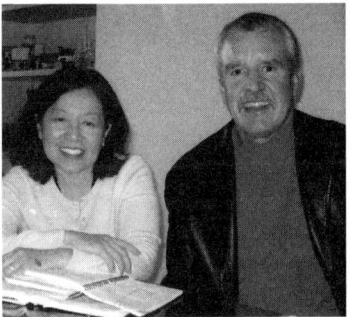

Aimee Hirabayashi, always my boss. Tom Bailey, a partner in my company.

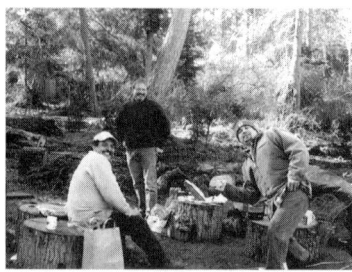

Mike, Ishmel and Gary working hard on
our property. What a crew.

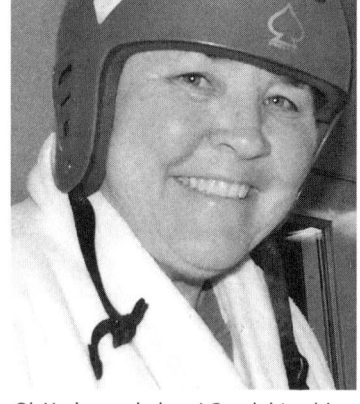

Oh Yeah... my helmet! Good thing blue
is my favorite color – my sweatpants
matched perfectly.

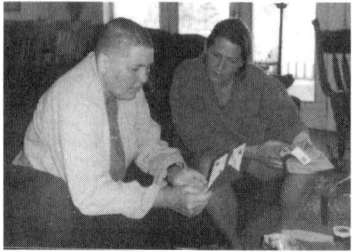

1st day home from Harborview
Hospital... Paula's birthday.
What a present!

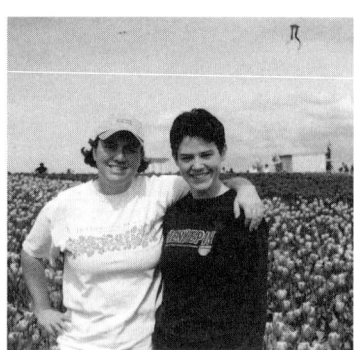

Lifesavers, Susan and Jenna tiptoeing
through the tulips in the Skagit Valley!

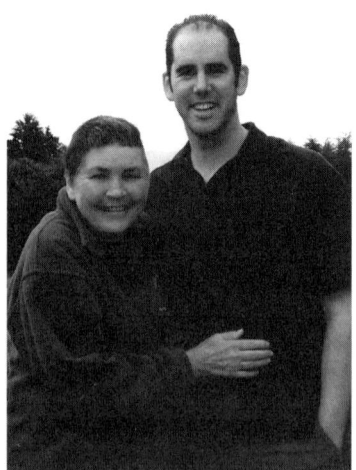

Wil Soholt, essential in my life, visited
from California in July 2007. My bone
was just recently put back in.
No more helmet.

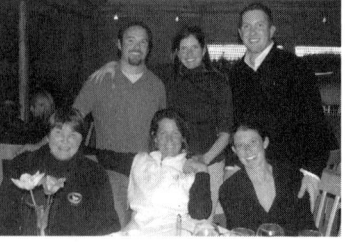

Celebration dinner with Kelly, Patrick,
Kris and Chad

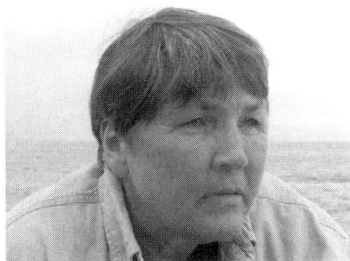

I love to think and solve serious concerns when looking at the ocean in Maui.

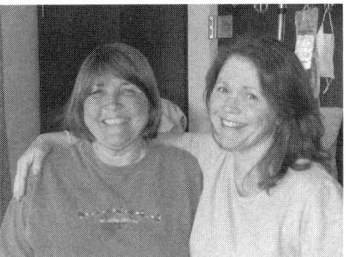

Getting ready for Session 1 of chemotherapy in Everett with my sister Dori by my side.

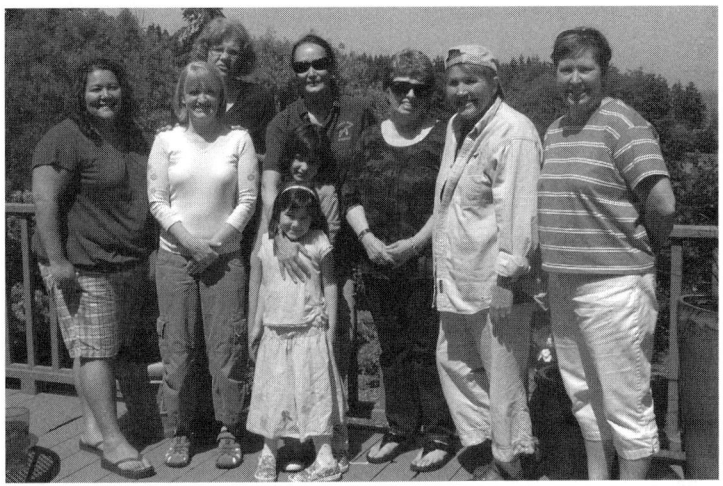

Celebration for surviving Session 1 of chemotherapy! Jasmine, Mary, Val, Kathy, Jane, me, Therese and Kathy's children Helen and Mary.

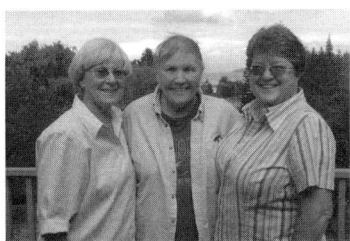

July 2009, Barb, Bonnie and I back home after Session 1. Lookin' good and waiting for the beauty pageant to call and let me know that I won!

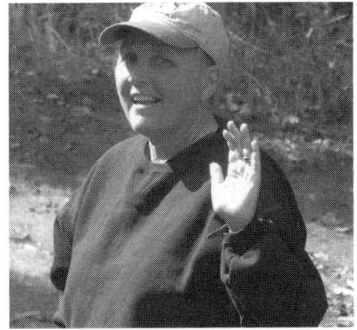

All my hair finally out… that didn't take long!

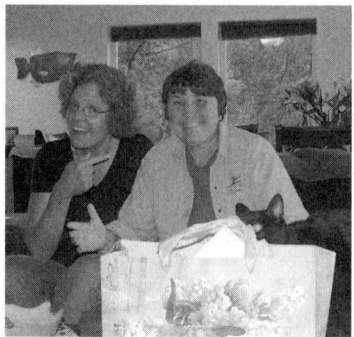

My birthday with Mary in
September 2010 – all smiles.

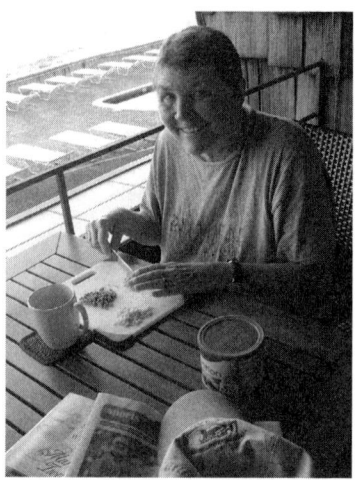

December 2009 feeding my birds
in Maui.

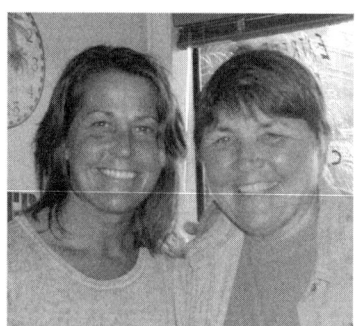

Maui 2007 – Didn't think I would ever
see it again.

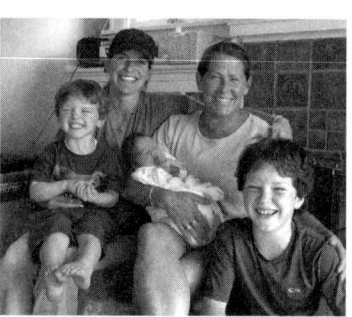

Paula with Kris and her boys.
Life is good.

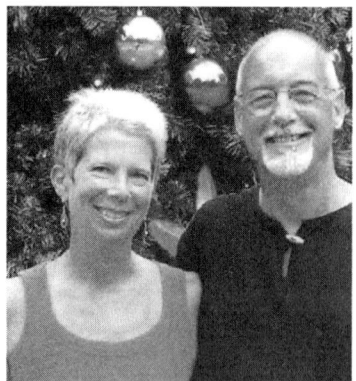

Long time friends Pamela Katims-
Steele and Patrick Steele – they have
walked with me each step of the way.

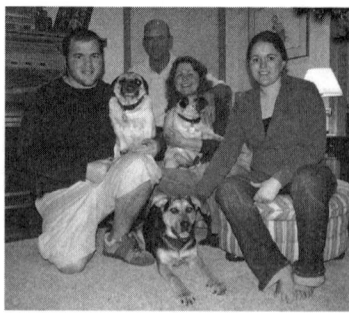

Daniel, John, Dori, Hilary and pups!

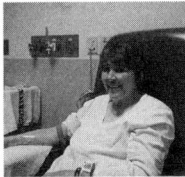

Getting prepared for my CAT scan at Harborview September 2010.

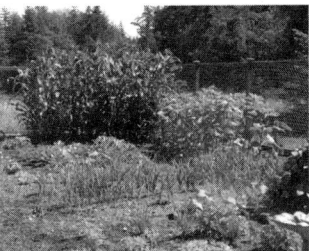

Our garden… Paula's place of peace.

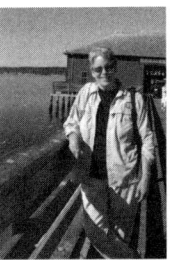

My longtime friend Nancy Brown enjoying the Coupeville Wharf.

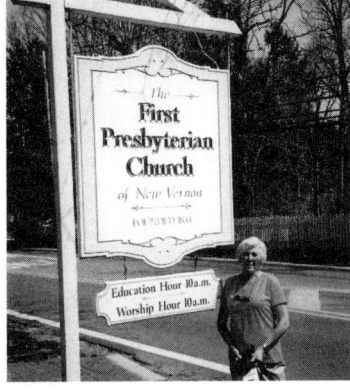

Paula's mom Bev – she wasn't afraid to sneak me out of the hospital!

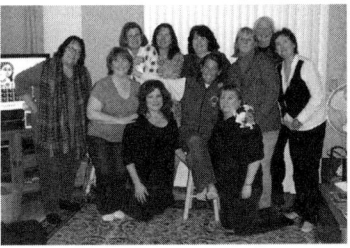

Paula spending time with her team – what an amazing group and support system for her.

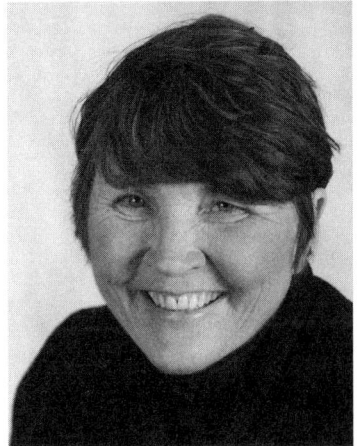

November 2010 – a little better than November 2009. Maybe the pageant will call this year.

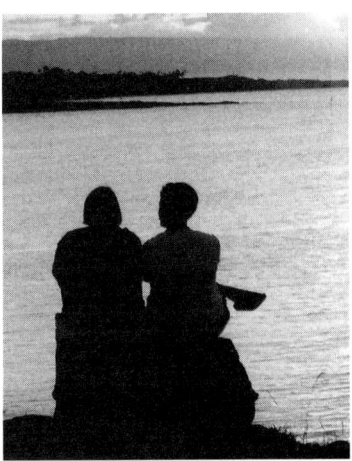

From here on out we will never forget to enjoy a beautiful sunset.

CHAPTER 11

◆ ◆ ◆

Are You Kidding Me?

I began feeling very tired at the end of March 2009. I had unexplained bruises all over my body and severe issues with my digestive system. I knew something was wrong but couldn't identify the source. I went to my local doctor who advised me to get a colonoscopy. I talked with the internist who scheduled the procedure. I felt that they hadn't done enough to eliminate other possible reasons for my exhaustion, because a blood test wasn't even going to be drawn. I put the colonoscopy off, hoping the symptoms would disappear. They didn't.

Paula and I were meeting Dori and her husband John in late May for lunch and shopping. It had been Paula's birthday the first part of April. I was excited to use this little trip as a means to get her the tennis shoes I had promised her for one of her birthday presents. The tennis shoes as a present, along with lots of other birthday presents, seemed so small and silly when she gave me life. How do I ever repay her for all the efforts she made?

We had a great day. I assumed it was fun for all because I was making my typical efforts to be funny. I was having trouble walking very fast, and I told Paula it was my shoes. I knew it wasn't my shoes, but I was frightened to try to find something wrong with my body, so I just walked slowly. I was glad when we finally reached home, because I felt exhausted.

The next day, Memorial Day 2009, I had no energy and could not wake up. I slept on the couch throughout the day while Paula worked in the yard. She continued to wake me up asking if I was OK. I would open my eyes, respond, and then fall back to sleep. About 9:00 p.m. Paula became concerned and called my best friend, Mary, who dashed over to our house. My temperature was 101. We headed for the ER at Whidbey General Hospital, the same hospital that saved me from dying of the brain aneurysm. Going to the ER was not something I ever signed up for. It meant significant trouble, and I had no idea what was happening to my body. I remembered I had trouble walking when I went shopping with Paula and claimed it was my shoes. Should I have been more honest? Maybe all of us should pay more attention to our bodies so we could sign up for doctor's appointments with our regular doctor during 8:00 a.m. to 5:00 p.m. I had done that in the past two months, but no solution had occurred, so the ER was my best option. The doctors are thorough, tests are readily available, and results are immediate. We often live because of this. Whidbey Hospital had saved my life over a brain aneurysm with their skill, resources, and the ability to get me to Harborview.

The ER doctor was very thorough and did extensive blood tests. They found that my counts were extremely low. The difference in my blood counts from November 2008, seven months prior, was incredible.

Type	November	May	Reference Ranges
White blood	6.2	1.20 L	4.8-10.8
Red blood	3.71 L	1.64 L	4.2- 5.4
ANC (neutrophils)	4.50	.1 L	1.5 -6.6
Platelets	197,000	20,000	140,000-450,000

We were able to get information about these four types of blood cells as they explained them to us. White blood cells fight infections where neutrophils, also called ANC, are a part of white blood cells. Their levels indicate the number of infection-fighting cells in your blood. These levels serve as an early warning. If those ANC numbers are low, your entire body is in jeopardy. Red blood cells carry oxygen and remove waste cells from the body's tissues. Platelets help the blood clot. When I thought about these and the differences between my November and May levels, I thought of ANC as "guards." The "guards" were able to help my body battle the infectious enemies who don't belong and need to be shown to the exit. The "guards" major job is eating the enemies so they cannot continue to attack. The enemies cannot be considered tasty.

There was definitely a problem. The ER doctor thought one possibility could be attributed to a medication I was taking for anxiety. That medication was stopped immediately, and an anti-diarrhea medication was prescribed. The ER doctor also indicated that leukemia could be the cause. I'd been going to so many doctors over the course of two years. Someone surely would have caught that! However, an appointment was set up for later that week to meet with a hematologist.

I continued to feel weak, and the bruising on my arms and legs along with a large bruise on my chest appeared from nowhere. The digestive issues had become "my running race," demanding a sprint to the bathroom. I lost that race fairly often.

Our meeting with Dr. Peter Y. Jiang M.D., Ph.D., Medical Oncology and Internal Medicine, occurred on Wednesday, May 27, 2009. After the blood tests were reviewed, he discussed the possibilities. He did not think the medication was responsible for the low blood counts and decided a bone marrow biopsy was needed for further analysis. That happened immediately.

I was ushered to a room and ordered to lie flat on my stomach. Some numbing medication was injected into my hip area. When the procedure began, it was similar to taking a wine bottle opener and manually screwing that into my hipbone. Thank God, I didn't remember the pain associated with the lumbar punctures I had at Harborview! I guess a brain injury is good for something. Dr. Jiang asked me to sign release forms to send my extra bone marrow to Fred Hutchinson Research Center. Sure, I thought. If they are consulting each other, that could help and support patients. I hoped it wasn't anemia, leukemia, or environmental issues. Even louder in my head was my desperate hope that all of this was something as simple as using the wrong medications.

I began to feel much better on Thursday. Paula was out working in the garden. She loves to be able to take the winter out of the garden and create the beginnings of a wonderful spring. She does all kinds of physical activities in the 2,400-foot garden. She creates perfect rows one after another. It is always touching to see amazing flowers and the variety of vegetables complementing each other. In the garden she feels peace. I worked vigorously on completing the brain aneurysm book. I felt excited that I could finish the book and share it with people by the end of the summer. Only I knew anxiety was again with me. That meant trouble, which I was soon to understand.

The call from Dr. Jiang came at 7:15 on Friday evening, earlier than expected. The news was devastating. I had been diagnosed with leukemia. He had this preliminary result, and the final diagnosis would be given on Monday. I was instructed to check into Providence Hospital in Everett, Washington at 1:00 p.m. the following Monday, June 1, 2009. By then he should have more information on the subtype of leukemia. I was expected to stay for 30 days to complete Session 1 of chemotherapy. The phone call lasted less than two minutes, and Paula and I were speechless. How could this be true? Let's see, I have struggled for two years to come back to myself. Now, with just two days' notice, I was supposed to accept a reality called hospital lock down. Maybe it's not called that, but that is clearly how it feels to me. How would I get out of this one? My heart ached, and I tried to look strong. As Paula wept uncontrollably, I let her know she was not alone this time. I can talk with her, I know who she is, and I can understand what she says. It may be even more difficult than the first bout of facing death, but at least the two of us will take this one on together.

◆ ◆ ◆

CHAPTER 12

2, 4, 6, 8....
Who Do We Appreciate?

Neither of us slept on Friday night, and Saturday was wrenching. Our hearts ached so much we were inconsolable. At least this time we had the weekend to prepare for the month ahead. We spent the day separate, both aching beyond imagination, unable to stop each other's pain. Could we go through this again? Did we have a choice?

When I thought about going to the hospital again, it was the sense that I had been through something terribly difficult the past two years, and I had worked so hard to come back to being myself. I still struggled with using the exact nouns I wanted in every sentence, and now I was facing something even more difficult. Was this my reward for having worked so hard?

Monday came too soon. I wasn't ready to leave the house, wondering if this was the last time I would be in my home. It was overwhelming. How does one say good-bye to their beloved animals? Take one last look at the yard and gardens? The pain was too deep for tears. I had never felt this before. I wondered if this is what Paula felt as she drove down the Island on her way to Harborview. Really, how much could one heart endure?

We were not alone at the meeting with Dr. Jiang for the final diagnosis. Kelly, Mary, Bev, and Paula waited impatiently with me for the news. I am sure this felt a little like their life in the ICU at Harborview. I was beginning to understand their fear because of the fear I was feeling. Mary had done her research on the different types of leukemia, their treatment protocols, and outcomes. When Dr. Jiang gave the news that I had APL (acute promyelocytic leukemia) Mary shouted, "Yeah!" I guess that was good news. He said, "APL is a rare form of leukemia with only fifteen hundred diagnoses a year in the United States. It also has a difficult treatment protocol, but a cure rate of 85%." I knew this would be a challenge, to say the least.

The treatment for APL consisted of one session of induction chemotherapy, another three sessions of chemotherapy, and two years of maintenance chemotherapy. As Dr. Jiang explained this it became clear that the induction chemotherapy was one of the most severe and the worst of the sessions for APL treatment. If I could make it through that round, my chances of recovery were high. But if my attempt failed, I would die.

I was put in a single room on the seventh floor of Providence Hospital. I was told I could not leave the floor and when outside the room I needed to wear a face-mask and plastic gloves to protect myself from germs. My blood counts were so low I was susceptible to catching anything. Kelly helped me prepare a sheet on *What Every Doctor and Nurse Should Know about Stephanie Haskins*. At last, I was famous.

What Every Doctor and Nurse Should Know About Stephanie Haskins June 1, 2009

1. I had a severe brain aneurysm February 2007. I am a miracle, I've been told. I have a shunt on the right side of my head. It is damaged by MRIs.
2. My doctor of choice in dealing with anything to do with my brain is Dr. Sekhar at Harborview.
3. I have had very severe diarrhea on and off the last month.
4. I have been taking blood pressure medicine to help with my shunt.
5. Sometimes I have trouble finding the right words when I am tired. Please be patient. I will get the right term eventually.

I greatly appreciated Kelly's help because I remembered like the brain aneurysm, I have a tendency to fight back. I may not be right, but I will stand up for what I believe about myself and others. People who worked with me in schools probably would remember that about me.

The nurses came to deliver morning pills and vitamins after I had been fed at 7:00 a.m. I remember thinking to myself that I doubted whether the vitamins would do any good. Every day I ordered breakfast, lunch, and dinner from Providence's menu. I thought they were pretending to be a restaurant, so I played along when I looked at their menu. I was trying to believe especially when I looked at their menu. There were pictures to accompany the menu items. The first one was beans in a bowl. The next one was a tiny little pizza with green peppers and tomatoes, the third one had muffins, and the last little square was coffee. Most interesting to me was the additional information on the title. It said, "At Your Request…Room Service Dining." Of course, I couldn't go anywhere else. It would be better for hospitals if patients could go out to dinner and they wouldn't have to worry about providing meals.

The induction therapy began on June 2 and was given on days 2, 4, 6, and 8. When you hear those numbers it brings back elementary school. It was "…2, 4, 6, 8, who do we appreciate?" Is it a poem? Is it a chant? In this case we did not appreciate those numbers. The goal of this round was to knock my blood count back to zero and wait for it to recover. I was given transfusions of red blood cells, protein, and platelets to increase my blood counts and help my body deal with the chemotherapy. The four injections of chemotherapy went well, and I felt fine. I wondered why I couldn't go home after day 8. I didn't realize it took time for the chemotherapy to wreak havoc on my body.

During the first two weeks, I would take walks around the floor in my mask and gloves accompanied by my medicine pole. At least I still had my hair. I liked walking down that hall because I could look out at homes across the street. One house was my favorite. There was a young mother with two children. She had a boy, a girl, and a fenced back yard. Every day was sunny, and the children would play in the sprinkler. There were clothes hanging on the line, and the house looked peaceful and happy. She looked like a perfect mom, and I felt a little sad that I would never hear her or stand next to her because I was sequestered on the seventh floor and the windows were sealed.

I was not allowed outside of the building. I don't think being kept from outside air helps patients get better. Here I was in a hospital where I could die, and I was not allowed to stand under the sky, walk on grass, or smell the air. I would never take the grass, sky, and air outside for granted again if I lived.

I noticed that other patients were not getting up and walking in the hallways. I remember thinking I was working hard and the only patient walking around. Why don't they too? The more that happened to me, and the sicker I became, the more I was like the other patients in the hospital. It became clear to me why patients didn't walk around. I even wondered if I would ever walk again.

We watched the Kentucky Derby. We had once watched a beautiful horse, Barbaro, win the derby. When he raced in the Preakness, he shattered his leg. The people who owned him tried to rescue him because he was so beautiful. They worked with him for about a year, but in the end, they put him to sleep at a very young age when he could have lived into his thirties. Maybe horse owners could figure out how to raise their horses so that racing doesn't cause their legs to shatter. It makes me think about people. Some die from cancer and others never get cancer, but I will continue to wish that no child or adult ever had to deal with cancer.

On June 9 and 10, I was still feeling OK. The doctor said the next five days would be crucial and would show the effects of the chemotherapy, and that I needed to just sit and wait. Bev brought me movies to watch, and I kept thinking I should just go home. On Thursday, June 11, they gave me a transfusion of red blood cells. My rear end started hurting and I had a fever. My temperature was 102, and I did not feel like going on my walk to see the house at the end of the hallway. Each day was worse. By June 14, I felt awful. It crossed my mind that I might die. How could I make it through the incredible journey of the aneurysm to die of leukemia?

The next day, June 15, the chemotherapy had taken its toll. Maybe they heard me talking about dying. My blood pressure dropped to 70/40 and the Emergency Medical

Team was called in. Doctors and nurses surrounded me, and Mary and Paula were kicked out of the room. It was weird to have all those people there. When I asked them why they were all in my room, they said they had to make sure I was going to be all right. It was frantic and I couldn't comprehend what was going on. All I wanted to do was sleep. They were getting prepared to insert a breathing tube when my blood pressure slowly began to increase. I don't think I could have handled that tube again.

My rear end was hurting, and a surgeon was called in for a consult. He immediately determined surgery would be required to remove an abscess. This was a tricky situation because my blood counts were low and I had no platelets to help my blood clot. The surgery took place on June 16 at 10:30 p.m. I came back to my room thinking death was just around the corner. My blood had difficulty clotting, and the next afternoon Paula rolled me over to discover I was lying in a large pool of blood. The doctors repacked the wound, and I waited to see if I could recover. I did.

I began losing my hair that had taken almost two years to grow back. My scars and shunt were beginning to show. Every morning when I looked in the mirror I had a re-minder of what I had already been through. Mary and I watched the movie *50 First Dates* a number of times. I loved the movie because it was about all the people who loved Drew Barrymore's character, a woman who had to start her life all over again each new day. People who loved her stood by her, took her hand, and shared her yesterdays as though they mattered. They did. I, too, couldn't remember what was said or done around me even if it happened only an hour earlier. Watching the movie reminded me, not only of the people in that movie, but of all the people who helped me survive with my broken brain. People make all the difference: people you love, who love you. They will support me again whether I have hair or not, whether we can visit or are told to be isolated, whether I am sick to the core, when fundamentally I'm not me. But, I am in there somewhere, and I want to come out again.

There are many differences between my two experiences. With my brain aneurysm, each day I improved and recovered. The leukemia was the opposite. Every day made me sicker, but at least my brain worked, and although I didn't like their TV, I could use the remote control and call the nurses if I needed something. Paula, Mary, Dori, and Bev took turns being at the hospital.

By June 20, the antibiotics and transfusions were beginning to work. Dr. Jiang said I could go home as soon as I had three consecutive days without a fever. I was beginning to feel better and began taking my walks again. Mary and I made a list of what I had already dealt with: fevers of 102, mouth sores, red raised rash, peeling lips, dry skin, no hair, diarrhea, swollen feet and ankles, crackle sounds in lungs, abscess under my arm, CT scan, dry/bloody nose, abscess surgery, and an allergic reaction to an antibiotic.

Wasn't that enough? Nope. It was time for another bone marrow biopsy on June 23. The results returned, and the cancer cells were gone. The chemotherapy had worked. Now I wondered if I could get out of having the other sessions of chemotherapy.

Finally, June 26, I began looking forward to going home. We were just waiting for my blood to recover and my fever to return to normal. I really wanted to go outside and actually be in charge of taking a first step and then a second and then a third, oh, yeah. It was hospital policy that no patients leave the hospital. However, we decided breaking the rules in this case would help my recovery. Paula made sure I was not wearing hospital clothes or a mask and to stay close. We ventured outside as if we were merely visitors. Family members continued to take me for walks, which was fabulous! The warm air, fragrant flowers, clouds, and that house! I had made it outside. I will always remember that feeling of joy and triumph. I began taking those secretive walks twice a day, and my strength returned. Breaking the rules helped in my recovery, and to this day I am glad we did it! Being outside was the answer to my recovery, and my blood counts began to increase.

On June 29, Dr. Jiang cleared me to go home. Paula and I had packed my belongings in big orange bags, just like Harborview. At least she only had to pack me up once this time! We returned home early that evening, and I was overcome with emotion as we drove down our driveway. I had made it.

◆ ◆ ◆

CHAPTER 13

Isolation

As I tried to come back from a brain aneurysm and struggled to survive leukemia, I thought about how I had built my life. Many of us do not spend time reviewing our lives until we face our own mortality. Now, I feel it is crucial to recognize every day, each day, because that is all we have for sure.

Coming home to recover from leukemia treatment involved a number of new rules. My interactions with people were minimal. I was very susceptible, and catching anything could send me back to the hospital or worse. The house was spotless and smelled of bleach. I spent the first three weeks of July recovering from that awful induction session. Paula spent much of her time cleaning, cooking healthy foods, and working outside. Luckily, the weather was beautiful, and I sat outside most days enjoying the warm weather, standing under the sky, walking on the grass, and smelling the air.

I returned to the hospital weekly for a blood check

and started to think about the next encounter that was coming. Dr. Jiang had a trip to China in July, where he volunteers to work with people who have no access to health care. He donates medical services for people with diabetes, high blood pressure, and other illnesses. Due to his schedule, I would not start Session 2 until July 20. It was difficult to imagine the months ahead and how involved and painful the process would be. I did not understand chemotherapy and the fact that it cannot and still does not separate healthy cells in your body from cancer cells. In my head, heart, and soul I feel like there is something wrong with our approach. Instead of doing things to eliminate only cancer, the use of chemotherapy also destroys our healthy cells. Chemotherapy kills them all.

On July 15, 2009, my blood counts recovered enough for me to hold a luncheon for friends and family. It was a beautiful day. I wore my hat to cover my baldhead, shunt, and scars. We celebrated that I was still living. Those summer days let me pretend I was actually ordinary. I knew that was not the case, but the thought was wonderful.

I continued to be very nervous about what would happen with Session 2. From the time I woke up in the morning until going to sleep, I was frightened. I did not want another stay in the hospital. I understood that Session 2 involved less chemotherapy, and Dr. Jiang was confident I would be able to remain at home. I did not have the same confidence.

Session 2 began on July 20 and involved four days of injections. We drove to the hospital on Whidbey Island each day for the hour-long treatment. After the four days of treatment, the waiting began. How would my body react? The description of the chemotherapy they used and the side effects indicated I would reach the low point, known as nadir, between days 10-15. Our last blood draw was July 20. The numbers were high, and I knew they would go down on the way to nadir. On August 3, day 14 of session 2, I knew my nadir had arrived, but I did not know the blood numbers. I thought I was feeling well enough to ride to Home Depot with Paula, wait in the car, and watch all the people who went into and out of the store. Then, however, I decided it would not hurt to go into the store as long as I did not touch anything. I wore gloves and a mask, my favorite new outfit, (okay, not really). I just wanted to get out. I was tired of thinking about my body and health 24 hours a day as an isolate, my new identity. I wanted an escape. We ran into Kelly inside the store, and she immediately gave me a lecture. She told me to be smart and make better decisions about my body. She reminded me of the serious ramifications this little trip could have on my health. She was right; I was wrong. Two days later, we had the usual Wednesday blood check. The results were exceptionally low. To check out of Providence at Everett the number of my ANC, or as I called them, my "guards," had to be at least .5. My "guards" were a mere .2. From that day on, I listened to Kelly and remained in isolation.

By August 12, 2009, my blood counts were going back up, particularly my "guards." They were very happy. When my "guards" are feeling better, I always know because it is an indicator of the body's ability to fight infections. We began to relax and enjoy the rest of the summer waiting for Session 3. It was great to have some time just being. Paula sat in the hot tub, worked in the garden, drove the mower, and played with her dog. We also grew some wonderful vegetables, corn, tomatoes, sweet onions, cabbage, and zucchini to name a few.

On the first day of Session 3, Monday, August 31, the oncology nurse reviewed the side effects of the new chemotherapy drug that would invade my body. It would be much larger and stronger. Would this cause another month-long stay in the hospital? I wasn't sure I could take it.

This session of chemotherapy was five days long ending on September 4, my birthday. The ONC nurses brought me a cupcake and sang happy birthday to me. These wonderful people do whatever they can to encourage people with cancer. I had mixed feelings about spending my birthday in a hospital while chemotherapy pumped through my body, but did I have a choice? What was worst of all was the waiting. Imagine going to a doctor to have him help you with a sore throat. You expect after the discussion and some medications you will gradually get better and over it. I go in and am feeling better but will have my system loaded with chemotherapy that makes me get sicker and sicker and sicker. Deaths happen because of this treatment. How can they expect patients to be hopeful when they are required to wait for chemotherapy to kill cancer, knowing that it also will kill your healthy cells? It is hard to be optimistic to say the least.

Paula returned to school just about the time my nadir hit for Session 3. We were both concerned that I would need support and decided to hire a retired nurse to spend the days with me at home. Sue was retired and lived nearby. She helped us out during my recovery from the aneurysm and was fabulous. She worked with Paula to administer my medication, take my temperature, bleach the house, and monitor my recovery. By September 10, I was not feeling well. Paula returned from school and checked my temperature, it was normal, but I sure did not feel normal. At 3:00 a.m. Paula found me standing in the living room upstairs, very unaware of my surroundings. My temperature had jumped to 103. She immediately called Mary and headed for the hospital. I was in the ICU at Whidbey General by 6:45 a.m. My "guards" were at zero, and I had pneumonia. I had lost my goal of staying home and this battle of chemotherapy.

I felt horrible but was glad to be on the island and not at the hospital in Everett. Paula would come to the hospital every morning before work and again after her work. Sue stayed with me throughout the day, and Mary came by daily. At least I had to look forward to something. The first few days I was very sick. I was very hot and nauseated. I threw up. When I began to get sick the nurses gave me medication intended to manage nausea. The nurses gave me the same antibiotic given to me at Providence that caused an allergic reaction. We wondered why the hospitals do not communicate with each other so reactions to various medicines, or mistakes, are not repeated.

The next two days they gave me various pills to address my symptoms. I threw up again on the second day. The doctors were trying to figure out what was causing all my pains and what to do. It was ironic to me that they thought what caused my pains was something other than the chemotherapy. Now how could that be since I did not have any of this until I received the chemotherapy? It was not that chemotherapy was an infection, but it was that chemotherapy destroyed my white cells along with other cells, which opened the door to any number of the enemies to my body. I could be upset and angry about a specific type of infection or getting pneumonia or throwing up when without the "so-called" help of chemotherapy my body could have protected me. I guess the trade off is life.

Bonnie Block's Reflection:

Hell, yes, the trade-off is LIFE! That is why they keep giving you the chemotherapy that causes such awful symptoms. I believe that you are alive because of the chemotherapy, not in-spite-of it. It would be terrific if the doctors could cure you without poisoning you. It would be great if they could identify the 15% who need additional poison. The fact is they cannot. I believe that many brilliant minds are out there right now trying to find cures or less-debilitating treatments for leukemia and other types of cancer. Until one of those things happens, I will continue to be thankful that chemotherapy was available to you.

I guess Bonnie had strong emotions on that point! I continued to have a high temperature and chills at night. I was feeling pain in a variety of places. I felt like nurses came in on a parade all day long. I would swallow something or there would be something in an intravenous bag dripping into my body. On the 16th, Dr. Jiang said I would need to stay in the hospital at least seven more days. They were clearly doing things that I would not be able to manage at home, even if I had a nurse. I received transfusions during this time to help my blood recover. The drugs were intended to help my body fight back from the chemotherapy.

Starting on September 17, I was gradually getting better. The pneumonia was gone and other infections had cleared up, but my "guards" were still at their lowest. My blood pressure was up to 180. That is significant because, as a result, of my brain aneurysm I was supposed to keep my blood pressure between 120–140. If my blood pressure is too high, it can damage the brain and cause a stroke, leading to my sudden death.

I remained in the hospital at Whidbey General until September 26, a total of 15 days. My body was having difficulty recovering because the more chemotherapy they put into your body, the harder it is to recover. My "guards" were still at the lowest, but Dr. Jiang felt it was safer for me to recover at home away from the many sick patients in the hospital. I might have laughed at the notion of the hospital being even sicker than I am. I just could not find it funny. After only two days at home, my "guards" had increased and were back to normal. Way to go "guards"!

I was glad to be back at home. I knew that Sue would be at my house every day until I got better. Paula would leave notes for Sue to read when she arrived, and then she would leave responses based on the day. As my body finally had the chance to recuperate, I felt I had gotten through the worst, Session 3. It was hard for me to understand that people who were in charge of medicine would be comfortable giving patient's things that are utterly brutal.

My blood finally began to recover by the middle of October. They did a bone marrow biopsy on October 21, and the result was great news--once again, no cancer. My blood counts were not great but improving. It was time to schedule the last session. Could I do it? The thought of more sessions produced uncontrollable fear in me again.

CHAPTER 14

◆ ◆ ◆

Knock Out!

Session 4 was only one injection and was administered on October 28. I really believed that it might be minor because it was only one shot, and I was going to have a month and a half to recover. As we did in the other sessions, we kept charts of my blood counts each week. By the third week, November 11, 2009, my ANC was down to .1. Clearly, my "guards" were not defending me. Even so, I wasn't worried because it was only the third week, which meant nadir had arrived. I had plenty of time to recover before departing for Maui on December 19. As we went from week to week, my blood kept going down even though the Session 4 dosage was the lightest. Instead of being mild and easy to get through, in fact, it was the opposite. Why would it ever be all right to knock the patient's blood out? This isn't a winning football game for me because my healthy cells were tackled and most were in fact, killed by the other team, chemotherapy. I was losing.

At our Wednesday meeting, December 2, 2009, Dr. Jiang said my blood counts needed to be higher in order for me to make the trip. It hurt my heart. Fear began to take over. I no longer had control of my trip to Maui, the one place I have always been able to go to find peace.

Even though I had a very low dosage, my body had been so assaulted my blood wasn't up to the last challenge. It's *Jeopardy* and the answer is, "chemotherapy, but not always." Can you come up with the question: "What kills cancer, but not you?" It shook me to the core. I had tried so hard and been through so much I wondered if I was not intended to live. I had trusted my doctor and followed all the directions, hoping that would be enough. Then it dawned on me. They don't know. They don't have a cure. They don't have a solution. They keep doing whatever they have been medically advised to do and despite, the individuality of each of us, they keep operating by following protocols that assume we are all the same. But we are in fact, just like kids in schools, individuals.

The following week at our December 9 meeting my "guards" had passed out. No power. This number is still way too low to make the trip. It had to be much higher. I was angry, frustrated, scared, but I had one more week before I would have to cancel Maui. I had developed a bad cold, and Dr. Jiang said that could be the problem. He told me to do things I do when I am trying to get over a cold. How could my blood counts increase that much in only seven days even if I was drinking lots or orange juice and keeping warm? Would that make any difference?

After a very stressful and anxiety filled week, we returned on December 16 for the final blood draw prior to our scheduled trip. My "guards" had gone up 160% and all I needed was 50% to be set free. My cold was over, and I was ecstatic that I was able to go to Maui!

When I got off the plane in Maui, I was so glad to see the palm trees, because they always indicate whether the trade winds are blowing. It is a sight that makes me feel free. The sound of the palms, the gentle wind, and the blue, blue, sky is peaceful. You can understand what's happening, whether it is pain or joy, if you have a vision that is just for you, seeing yourself clearly. As we drove toward the place we stay, I was overwhelmed with emotion again. This time it was happiness, and I could not control the tears. Two weeks of peace. No blood draws or bleach wipes, at last, a time out.

Time moves much slower. When I am in Washington, time seems like it is racing through the hours to get to the next day. In Maui things are quiet, and I can observe almost every hour because it goes slowly enough for me to keep up with it. I always know that I have to go back home when Maui time starts to seem like it is racing through the hours. Maui doesn't change, I do.

In the winter there are amazing humpback whales that interact with one another in the ocean. I go snorkeling and see all the wonderful, colorful fish off several beautiful beaches. Miniature crabs run from one hole to another. Large turtles feed themselves off the coral just a few feet out from our place. I set up a little bird feeding spot on the lanai and greet them each day with finely chopped nuts. The various birds express themselves individually and say hello to me while enjoying the snack. They compete with each other as to who gets to take bites first. I put out enough for them so that even if there is a mini competition its fairly gentle because they all know there is enough for each of them. They wait for me to do the same thing the next day. That's kind of how people can behave.

The sunsets are stunning as they go slowly into the ocean and their last beautiful multiple colors fill the sky above the ocean. It is as if it really will never leave you. There are many places to visit. Lahaina is a wonderful little town with lots of shops. Wailuku and Kahului are older larger towns near the airport. The towns are great, with interesting stores. They are so open and inviting that I want to jump out and go in and visit. Up Country Maui has amazing views of the ocean and great farms. I also love the names. They reflect the people who were here long before any others began to dance toward these islands.

What helped me over the past three years were the songs by Israel Kamakawlwo'ole, or IZ. He was a true Hawaiian. His words touched me then and continue to today. The words he combined from "Over the Rainbow" and "What a Wonderful World" are truly amazing and put life in perspective.

My favorite words…

"Oh, somewhere over the rainbow, blue birds fly, And the dreams that you dreamed of, dreams really do come true, and I hear babies cry, and I watch them grow, They'll learn much more than we'll ever know, And I think to myself, What a wonderful world!"

Truly, it is a wonderful world we live in. Visiting Maui helped me see me. If I could be peaceful in Maui and be honest with myself, I would be able to go home and be strong. I wanted to meet the challenge of leukemia. You have to know yourself well enough to recognize what is needed as you take each step toward regaining your life.

The day we left I was exceptionally sad. I didn't want to return and go through any more. I knew the chemotherapy sessions were complete, but two more years of chemotherapy weekly injections and blood draws? Why couldn't it just be over?

We returned to meet with Dr. Jiang on January 6. When I looked at my blood count report, I was totally surprised. The numbers were generally higher than they had been. Maui was the answer! Two days later, I had another bone marrow biopsy. This one was extremely painful, more so than the previous biopsies. It was frightening to imagine that I had gone through chemotherapy starting June 1, 2009, and after induction therapy, the June 23 biopsy indicated the leukemia was gone. My next biopsy was on October 21, 2009, when I had completed Session 2 and Session 3. This showed CMR, complete molecular remission, and showed zero cancer cells out of a million cells. Again, clear of leukemia. The January 8, 2010, biopsy results came back and, once again, no leukemia. At this point I really began to wonder why it was necessary to continue injecting chemotherapy when each time they check, my cancer is gone. It makes no sense to me.

Session 5 was to start January 20, 2010. The idea of facing weekly and daily chemotherapy for maintenance was not attractive. I outlined the questions I had about Session 5 and the maintenance treatment. I put together questions; I have done that all my life. If I don't understand I always ask questions that I have written or typed so that I have the answers and am clear. Dr. Jiang wanted to follow the protocol, so they would be giving me two different chemotherapies. One of them is an injection into the fatty tissue of the hip. My dose was to be 30mg. once a week. The other chemotherapy was two pills that I would take each night for a total of 100mg. Dr. Jiang's expectation was that chemotherapy would not affect my blood counts too much. When I looked at my questions and Mary's notes, I still had one fundamental question. Do we look at patients as individuals and recognize that what works for one doesn't necessarily work for another?

Dr. Jiang assigned me the recommended maintenance protocol for my APL leukemia. He indicated that maintenance was the final step of permanently eradicating APL for the rest of my life. He told us that studies indicated that APL people who did not do maintenance had the danger of its coming back. Although 85% would never get it again, the fact was that 15% could. He said maintenance was like getting an insurance policy. When I thought about it later, I realized that maintenance is nothing like an ordinary insurance policy. For me to face having chemotherapy for one to two more years didn't sound at all like good insurance, especially since I could be in the 85% group. Why does this happen? Why do medical people support and choose to give chemotherapy treatment to people who don't need it? Why should we stand for putting something in us that absolutely hurts our body cells? If we had curing cancer as our first and foremost goal that is supported by all of us, maybe these discussions and practices could end.

I wasn't overly concerned about my body's ability to respond to the chemotherapy because the protocol was a mild dosage. However, my body did not respond as expected. I decided this was the time to do things I could do while I was alive. I think that we sometimes don't do things we would enjoy because we are concerned about our daily lives, and we tell ourselves there will always be another time. The reality for me now is that I can only count on the day I wake up, and if I don't do with it what I'd like, that day is gone forever.

When I found out the Bette Midler show in Las Vegas was coming to an end, I knew I had to attend. Her energy, performance, focus, laughter, and tears presented through her talent always cheered me up, made me think, and made me feel that I could take on things to make my world a better place. I love her shows. She has been great in movies, and she represented all of us in her song and words to Johnny Carson on his last show. I think that of all the things she has done in her career the best is seeing her on stage where she interacts and connects with the audience. She makes me and millions of others feel wonderful. I could touch the stage from my seat, and Bette was just five feet away from me. I was so grateful to be alive and to do something that involved going out among other people. Thanks again, Bette Midler.

When Mary and I got back to the room after Bette's show, I did not feel very well. I was exhausted because I had eight months of dealing with chemotherapy at home and in two long stays in the hospital. I soon discovered that the maintenance wasn't mild for me at all. We had to catch the plane back home the next morning. I started getting really sick around five in the morning. I took the pills that I had successfully used at other times. We got on the plane and for the first time in my life, I had first class seats in the front of the plane. They have bigger seats and a separate bathroom. The flight was only two and a half hours but I had spent much of it in the bathroom. I was scared. Why was I having such an adverse reaction to the chemotherapy? Wasn't everything supposed to be fine? What was going on? I started thinking about everything I had been through the past three years. Surgeries, medications, injections – was my body shutting down?

When I got home I thought about how much Bette Midler had influenced me. I know that people who love music have favorite singers who make their lives better. I had never sent a thank you note to Bette about how much her incredible work had helped me during my life. I tried to tell her how I felt about her in a telegram that I wrote and sent the day I was back at home. I hope that all of us take a few minutes to say thank you directly to the people who enrich our lives.

I still felt sick when I got back home, but I was determined to thank Bette and sent her that telegram. It was Wednesday, January 27, 2010, my least favorite day of the week because that is the day I go to the hospital. I typed up a page of my daily symptoms to share with Dr. Jiang. "I have felt lousy every day. I can't really go anywhere, because I can't be away from a bathroom. If I take the pill, I feel bloated, and my whole body is stuffed and strained. It aches and I feel bad all over. If I don't take a pill, I cannot control how often I'm in the bathroom. This is not working for me. That's what happened in May of last year, and that led us to my leukemia diagnosis. Maybe it has gotten worse because I now have more of the chemotherapy in my body. Maybe my body just can't take any more."

I had nine different medicines to take daily. He suggested that I stop one and put it off for three months. The plan then was to take the daily pills and the weekly shot. I continued to feel miserable and was fighting low blood counts and digestive issues. At the February 17 meeting, Dr. Jiang said to reduce the pills from two tablets to one and a half and I would not get a shot that day. By the meeting on February 24, Dr. Jiang decided to stop all chemotherapy both the shots and pills. My blood numbers kept going down significantly. It was obvious to me that my body couldn't handle any more. In the next three or four days I started to feel better. I decided I was done with the chemotherapy and hoped I was in the 85% group.

Another concern was the bone marrow report from January 8. Although there were no leukemia cancer cells, the biopsy did report an abnormality on a different set of chromosomes. This didn't concern me at the time; I was concerned about the leukemia cells. However, this news was devastating to Paula and more frightening than cancer. She couldn't understand what was happening to my blood and thought it may be related to the amount of chemotherapy I had received. Paula's fear had caused her to ask many questions about the different set of chromosomes that were reported. She had talked with the ONC (oncology) nurses in January who had given her an overview of what that revealed. The chromosomes cited could be part of a syndrome called MDS. That abnormality was pointing towards a condition that cannot be treated. The bone marrow is not functioning, and medical support is providing patients with borrowed white blood cells, red blood cells, and platelets but ultimately, those supports cannot overcome the loss of a healthy bone marrow. Depending upon each person's body, MDS can result in death in less than a year.

Dr. Jiang decided it was time to send me to a specialist in Seattle. He recommended Dr. Estey, a specialist on APL. This recommendation by Dr. Jiang took courage, honesty, and understanding. He has vast knowledge as a result of the research portion of his career and tremendous listening sensitivity to each patient he supports. I think he is a wonderful doctor and is the kind of doctor who truly makes differences in peoples' lives. Others can definitely learn from him.

On March 9, 2010, Paula, Mary, and I went together to the Seattle Cancer Care Alliance. The building near Lake Union was beautiful. I would discuss the meeting in Seattle with Dr. Jiang the next day.

We listened to Dr. Estey, and he permitted us to tape our discussion. I was uncomfortable with the meeting because Dr. Estey was providing options. My dad made a living by selling to others. When I was young, my dad would go over various techniques to encourage and persuade people to buy his product. He did very well, and what I learned from him stayed with me. I felt that at the beginning of the meeting Dr. Estey was selling a method labeled arsenic. His presentation set me up to do more treatments and spend more money on health charges, when 85% of APL patients have been through chemotherapy sessions and have been successful at eliminating leukemia. When will there be a protocol and a policy developed where doctors identify the 85% who are free of cancer and will not relapse and focus specifically on the 15% who need additional treatment? What worries me is that even if patients have won the cancer battle, they continue having things put into their bodies that would never be a choice. How is it okay to continue to put chemotherapy into people who have shown they don't need it? Isn't it time that doctors and hospitals use medicines based on each individual's needs? Luckily, Dr. Jiang recognized this and changed the protocol that would support me.

When we left after our meeting with Dr. Estey, we headed back and stopped to have lunch at Chandler's Crab House on Lake Union. I was ecstatic! Dr. Estey had agreed with Dr. Jiang, no more maintenance chemotherapy! I ordered the oysters and loved them. My blood was too low to eat raw food but I didn't even think about it for the first time in nine months. What is ironic about this situation is the fact that the new issue of MDS didn't even register with me. I didn't remember his talking about it. Paula, on the other hand, was sick to her stomach. Her fear over the past two months was confirmed. This abnormality is serious. All we could do was wait to see the April bone marrow biopsy results.

This reminded me of my mom. She was diagnosed with esophageal cancer, and one day I went with her to her doctor's appointment. The doctor showed us an x-ray picture of her throat. When I saw it, I could hardly believe it. I stared at it. The bottom half of her throat was totally covered and appeared to be under a massive glob of cancer cells. I kept looking at it and my brain raced, thinking about my mom. I turned around and looked at her. She smiled her great smile at me. Smiling is how she got through life. I asked her what she thought about the x-ray and what she saw. She told me she couldn't see anything that would prevent her being alive. I remember saying that was good. She smiled again. Later she was in another room, and I talked to the doctor. I told the doctor I thought the x-ray looked horrific; what does it mean? The Doctor told me it was very serious and hoped that the radiation would provide some room in her throat so in her last few months she would be able to swallow. The doctor said she wasn't sure that could happen but she was going to try. She said if the treatment worked, my mother could live a few more months, perhaps up to six. If nothing was done, she had a few weeks to live. The radiation gave my mother not just a few months but five more years. She never did see the cancer cells on her throat just as I hadn't heard Dr. Estey discuss the abnormality and the possibility my bone marrow was wrecked. I had seen my mother's x-ray with clarity, and Paula heard Dr. Estey's concern that I may have MDS. I wonder if the patients see and hear only what they need to in order to keep their hopes alive.

CHAPTER 15

◆ ◆ ◆

Light at the End of the Tunnel

April finally arrived, and it was time for the long-awaited results. I had the biopsy procedure at Providence Medical Center in Everett on April 21. The procedure went smoothly, and the pain was minimal. Maybe this was a sign that the bone marrow was really working! Our appointment for the results was scheduled for Wednesday, April 28. I noticed that Paula was not sleeping well and seemed extremely anxious. I had no idea that she was preparing herself for the worst. The result of this biopsy could potentially confirm MDS.

On April 28, we got to the hospital early hoping to be seen earlier than scheduled. No luck. They were running unusually late that afternoon, and after an hour of waiting, I was ushered in and my blood drawn. Now the real wait began. I sat patiently in my recliner chair, reviewing the questions I had for Dr. Jiang. Paula was pacing anxiously and could not sit down or be consoled. She decided to sneak a peek at my chart hoping to find the

Pathology Report on my bone marrow biopsy. Suddenly, she shrieked with joy. No cancer! It took only a second for her to realize that she was looking at the January biopsy results. She was visibly shaken and frantic. She soon left to find information about the report. After nearly four months, she could not wait any longer. She needed to know the news.

Finally after two hours of waiting, Dr. Jiang appeared. My blood report came back, and my counts were strong. My platelets had gone up significantly in just a week, and the rest of my counts were stable. However, there was no news from the Pathology Report. Where was the report? Why hadn't it come back yet? Did it indicate MDS? While Dr. Jiang left to call the Pathologist at Providence Medical Center for the results, I thought Paula would crawl out of her skin. Dr. Jiang returned a few minutes later with the report in his hand. His face showed no indication of the results. A simple smile or furrowed brow would have said it all. Without emotion, he informed us that again, I was cancer-free. The bone marrow biopsy was free of leukemia cells. Next, with a big smile on his face, he shared the most amazing news of all the abnormal chromosomal growth had disappeared, and there was no MDS! It was over. We had won this battle too. As the news settled in, tears of joy began flowing. We couldn't believe it and wondered where that growth had gone or if it had been there at all! I guess we will never know the answer to that question. What we were given was the gift of time. We had time to live our lives without the worry of blood draws or biopsy results. But, how does a person do that after spending nearly three years battling a brain aneurysm and cancer? Maybe it is just time, time to reflect and begin trusting life again.

As summer approached, I slowly began trusting in life as each month my blood counts increased to within normal ranges and I felt healthy. In July, I enjoyed nearly three weeks on Maui. I thought maybe I would be healthy and live without any other major medical challenges. The remainder of the summer was spent completing this book. I decided it was essential to get both Dr. Sekhar and Dr. Jiang to sign release statements in order to publish their materials. It was also time for a routine CTA scan of my brain. I made an appointment with Dr. Sekhar and looked forward to seeing him after nearly two years. On September 22 Paula, Mary, and I headed for Harborview. It was a beautiful sunny day and our moods reflected the weather. It was so nice driving to Harborview for a test and nothing serious. After we arrived, I had my CTA (Angio) completed on the first floor. During the procedure, Mary and Paula were able to sit with the radiologist, and he gave them a play by play on the procedure. Harborview is wonderfully inclusive to allow family and friends into the room. After the procedure, Paula joked with me that I might hear rap music in my head for a day after the CTA scan. I let her know that it was not rap music I heard but my mother's voice. I had never heard her before, and I was emotional. I heard her say, "It is not time for you to come." It was as if she was inside my head and the message was loud and clear. I was perplexed to hear her now…what did it mean? I soon let the thought go as we went to visit the Neuro Specialty Floor to visit Queenie. As we approached, it was obviously an area that was under construction. Paula found the spot where I had fallen and put a two-foot hole in the wall. Along came Shayne Pitt, the carpenter who remembered repairing the hole. We had a few laughs and I took a picture with Shayne in front of the repaired hole. Queenie was not working that day, so we headed over for my appointment with Dr. Sekhar.

We again waited patiently for our appointment, with no fear of the outcome at all. This was a celebration and a time to thank Dr. Sekhar and share the book with him. After some time, a colleague of Dr. Sekhar entered the room and asked me the routine questions. He asked me if I had any residual symptoms from the brain aneurysm surgery and I answered, "Yes, fear." He asked if I had any other neurological symptoms like vision or walking, numbness or headaches. I answered, "No, I am way too tuned into what my body does, and any changes scare me." At that point, he compared the 2007 scan with the 2010 scan. Immediately, I sensed concern in Paula's voice as she asked him if the news was good. He then showed us an abnormality in the new scan and proceeded to explain that it was either another brain aneurysm, or cancer that had spread to the brain. In utter disbelief I ran out of the room and into the bathroom. I couldn't breathe. How could this be true? Did I hear him correctly? Paula and Mary asked Dr. Sekhar to come immediately. As I regained some composure, I reentered the room only to hear the same news from him. The scan showed a mass, and it was highly probable to be an aneurysm. Dr. Sekhar explained that it looked like a type of aneurysm that would require the vessel to be bypassed and connected to another vessel, as it contained its own blood supply. This diagnosis meant another major surgery, helmet, missing bone and long recovery. Paula asked if there was any good news or any chance it could be something else. The good news was there was an 80% chance it could be fixed and he doubted it was cancer. He would give us no more information until I had the complete angiogram, a test that would show exactly what we were dealing with. We made the appointment for Friday, September 24, two days away.

We left the hospital in shock. This news was unbelievable. How much can one person take? My brain could not stop. I felt so guilty for what this would do to my friends and family who had taken care of me. It was my turn to take care of them. The next day was as excruciating as the day I found out I had leukemia. I could not think straight and yet still had to pick up medication for the cerebral angiogram, get my shunt port flushed and be prepared to have brain surgery. I made many phone calls to rally friends and family once more to assist Paula to ensure she could remain in her job at school. I had the house and animals covered and spent the day too scared to cry. I wondered if it was worth it. Could my body take it? I was just beginning to trust life again. That trust was shattered in seconds. Could it ever be rebuilt?

On Friday, Mary and I left bright and early for a 9:00 a.m. appointment. The procedure is not painful but required me to lie flat for six hours to ensure clotting of the femoral artery. I slept the night prior and felt a sense of relief knowing I would have answers by the end of the day and not have to spend one more night wondering about the future. It was great to have Mary with me. She has such a positive outlook, and she truly believed there was a mistake in the scan, because no way could this be true. I wanted to believe in Mary's optimism, but Dr. Sekhar's words would not leave my head.

After much preparation, the procedure went smoothly. As the procedure was ending, I asked the radiologist for the results. He told me Dr. Sekhar would be the one to read the tests results to me. I became frantic knowing he knew what the test showed and began crying. I explained what the past three years had entailed for me and said I could not wait for Dr. Sekhar, I needed to know now. He responded that he felt comfortable sharing with me that it looked like a mass of calcium that required no surgery or treatment. He immediately followed up with the fact that Dr. Sekhar would have the final say, but it did not look serious to him. I could not believe it! I screamed and continued to say, "Thank you, thank you, thank you, thank you...you don't know what this means to me!" I was wheeled back to the recovery room and had to wait nearly an hour for Mary to return from getting food to share the news. When she arrived with a turkey sandwich, I told her it looked like we may have dodged another bullet and explained the radiologist's initial analysis. We were elated but awaited Dr. Sekhar's final word.

About 5:00 p.m., Dr. Sekhar arrived and confirmed the radiologist's analysis. It was calcification and there was no treatment needed. He told me that someone was definitely looking out for me! I am beginning to wonder if someone does these things to remind me that I have to stay focused and get this information out to people through a book and a Website. I am now staying focused, and if something comes up again, I would prefer it if I could be told quickly and avoid being scared to death. By anticipation, we called family and friends to share the great news. On the trip home, I remembered my mom's words in my head just two days before, "It isn't time for you to come." I now understood what she meant. It was time to build trust in life again.

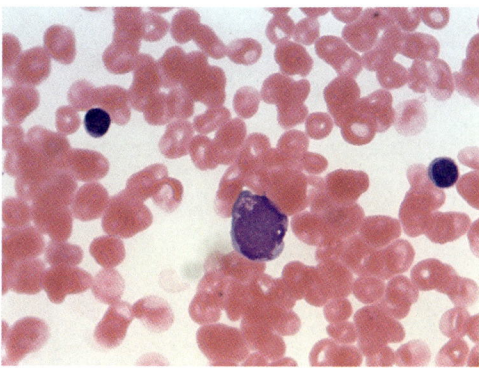

photo 1: blast and 2 lymphocytes for size comparison

The red "apple" like cells are red blood cells that carry oxygen around for the body. They were low in numbers, which explained your exhaustion before the bone marrow biopsy. The small blue cells are part of the "guards" cells called lymphocyte (the ANC was not present in this photo because there were so few of them). The large blue cell is the bad "guy," so called blast or APL cell. As you can see, it is large in size, vicious looking and there were many of them in the marrow. That is why they were "strong" and beating up your other smaller "good cells." They were the dominant cells then. That is why the chemotherapy needed to be stronger to suppress them and level the "field" for the smaller good cells to come back and take hold.

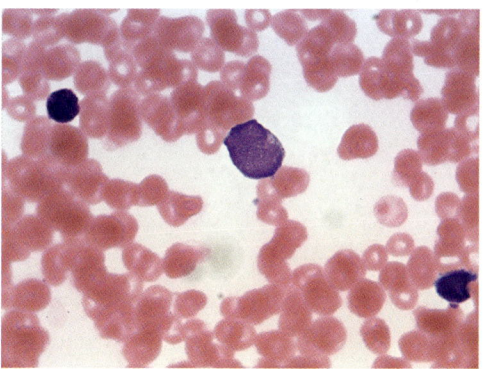

photo 2: blast with fine granules

This picture further explains the special feature of the large blue APL cell. It has fine blue granules like "salt-pepper." Each granule is like a bag with special chemicals in it. When the bag broke and chemical released, serious bleeding, called DIC (disseminated intravesicular coagulopathy), happens. With your history of brain aneurysm, these granules were the doctor's "nightmare" or "stress" during the first week, which I did not burden you all, and that was the reason you received the "protein" or plasma transfusion.

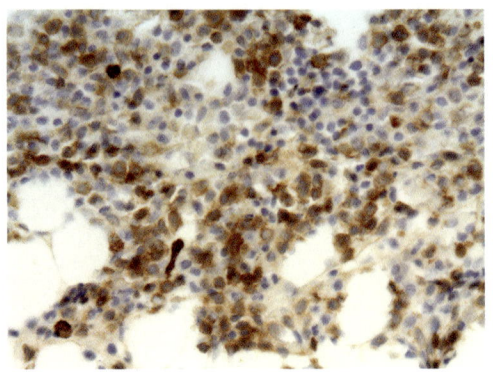

photo 3: CD 117 immunostain

The brown cells are marking positively and are the blasts.

◆ ◆ ◆

CHAPTER 16

Lessons Learned

This experience has changed me forever and amazingly enough, in a positive way. I was always focused as a teacher, principal, and consultant to do everything possible to help every child be successful. I was always in a hurry because of the numerous tasks to complete each day. What I learned through these experiences is that I had not taken the time to observe the world around me. I learned what a tremendous loss it is when we don't take time to acknowledge ourselves and the wonderful things that surround us.

When I moved to Whidbey seven years ago, I didn't notice the flowers, birds, or the other animals. Paula put up a feeder for hummingbirds each year. As a result of the struggle I had after the brain aneurysm, I couldn't remember their names and instead called them humdingers. Their behaviors gave me hope. How the male humdingers would dance to attract a female. How the feeder has one humdinger that thinks it is his own. Most humdingers leave each year, but some stay year round. When the humdingers return in the spring, it's as if they knock on the door to let me know they are ready again in the new spring. Instead of one feeder, we now have five feeders, and the humdingers visit them many times each day. I now notice and feed the squirrels, chipmunks, bunnies, and many other birds. These animals are a vital part of my day. I talk to them, feed them, and make sure they are OK. I would not recommend almost dying twice in order to learn this lesson.

I have been forced to ask the question, "What is life?" I realize that the most valuable lesson I have learned is to embrace what society refers to as the "little things." They are not "little things" … they are what matter. We spend too much of our time focused on work, problems, and accomplishing tasks. Life is the small, everyday experiences to which we don't pay enough attention. If that is all I have to worry about, then life is indeed wonderful!

Thank you for reading our story. We hope it touched your life. Remember each day to appreciate the "little things."

P.S. Together We're Better!

Throughout both traumatic ordeals, a brain aneurysm and leukemia, I learned a great deal about medical procedures. I also learned a great deal about nurses, doctors, and specifically, patients. I became aware of pharmaceutical companies, the medications they produce, and the amount of money made on these products. Is it any wonder there are not enough resources going to finding a cure for cancer?

The people who have supported me through the two-year challenge by the brain aneurysm have told me they are amazed at how articulate I am. So many friends were exceptionally supportive to ensure my progress. We need hospitals to coordinate rather than compete. The Mayo Clinic has a new method called analytics technology. Mayo and IBM collaborated and came up with what is called Medical Imagining Informatics Innovation Center, which has proved to be 95% accurate rate in detecting aneurysms. Many say I am a miracle because I managed to live and recover from a brain aneurism when the majority of people who have this die. This latest collaboration of Mayo and IBM has created a way of checking people prior to their brain aneurysm's rupturing. This is in the clinical trials now, and we hope that it will move toward commercialism and have this treatment available to hospitals all around the United States.

It feels fabulous to me to know that it is possible to prevent people from going through what I did and keeping people from dying from a brain aneurysm. Thank you Mayo Clinic and IBM for the efforts you have made.

Until this is available everywhere in this country, you need to know a basic fact. If you have a severe headache, one you have never had, you and your loved ones must connect immediately with hospital emergency. You must know and access the hospital that is most equipped to deal with this immediately and give you the best chance of surviving.

The second challenge of another year following the brain aneurysm, APL leukemia, also enhanced my knowledge of medical and health issues. Literally, millions have leukemia and cancer. Those numbers are bad but are even worse when you see that children are included in the devastation of cancer and leukemia.

I am grateful that chemotherapy is available and that it fights cancer. It has been successful in treating cancer for millions of people. The problem is what happens to us when chemotherapy is injected into our bodies? The following quote is from Scott Hamilton's website. Scott, an American figure skater and an Olympic Gold Medalist, has taken on the responsibility of addressing cancer and defining various aspects of this website called Chemocare.com.

Chemotherapy is most effective killing cells that are rapidly dividing. Unfortunately, chemotherapy does not know the difference between the cancerous cells and the normal cells. The "normal" cells will grow back and be healthy, but in the meantime, side effects occur. The "normal" cells that are most commonly affected by chemotherapy are blood cells in the mouth, stomach and bowel, and the hair follicles; resulting in low blood counts, mouth sores, nausea, diarrhea, and/or hair loss. Different drugs may affect different parts of the body.

I wonder what would happen if all us got together to encourage and support those who are looking for ways to eliminate chemotherapies that still, after more than fifty years, have not found medications that address cancer and does not damage normal healthy cells. Some are saying now that what is done to your body through the use of chemotherapy may cure cancer in the short run but may also make people more vulnerable for other cancers in the long run.

We can work together to pull resources and address the total prevention of brain aneurysms and the prevention of cancer. There are around 80 million Baby Boomers. So, Baby Boomers, it's time we get together to make changes in this country that will have positive results for all of us, especially for our children and grand children. I have given donations to heart, cancer, and other large organizations every year. I usually give to each one. I don't know what they are doing; they don't survey me or call me and ask what I would like, I just donate like everyone else. Some have said that medical people were identifying cancer as far back as 1845. I totally believe if we all stood up together and together we said we want cancer eliminated and prevented now, we would meet that challenge.

I am not writing this book to make money. I am writing this to help save lives, to help people. Proceeds from this book will be directed to the most effective and successful research on eliminating both cancer and aneurysms. Finally, this isn't about politics. It is not important how you vote or your party affiliation. What matters is that we stand together and use our small contributions to voice and influence the changes that need to occur for us all.

Please visit our website
www.beataneurysmandleukemia.com
for more information and remember...

Together We're Better.

Thank You

We wish to acknowledge and recognize each person who helped us. Together your efforts taught us to recognize how unique and wonderful people truly are. People did a variety of tasks to show their support. Some sent emails and cards, others took care of the house and animals, while many others visited, cooked meals, or made phone calls. Thank you all. Printing the names is a small token and we will forever be working on "paying it forward." If we have forgotten a name, we humbly apologize.

Family:

Julie Haskins, Michael Haskins, Suzy Haskins; Dori and John Mosich, Daniel Mosich, Hilary Mosich; Bev Seaman; Sarah, Hannah and Josie Bear; David, Amy, Ellie and Ben Seaman; Sharon, Leaf, Caleb and Anna Van Boven; and Wil Soholt.

Friends who read, assisted with the development, and helped edit this book:

Bonnie Block, Nancy Brown, Linda Clay, Barb Greenlee, Mary Heck, Pamela Katims Steele.

Kristin Zwiers Photography:

A special thanks to our friend Kris for her patience, talent, and consistent support of this project in organizing and presenting the photographs in this book.

Crescent Harbor Elementary Family:

There are no words to express my gratitude. You are the most amazing staff anyone could imagine working with. Your constant kind words, thoughts and love made the difference for me every day. No matter what the future brings, my heart belongs to you all.

Friends and Supporters:

Tunde Akunyun, Sharon Anderson, Tom Bailey, Walt Bankowski, Deanna Barret, Linda Bartling, Gene Beall, Terry Bergeson, Colette Blangy, Jenna Brown, Susan Buntich, Shirley and Dave Burbank, Bi Hoa Caldwell, Nina Chambers, Rebecca Ching, Jeff and Susie Clark, Kelly, Patrick, Addie and Mylah Cleary, Gail Cleveland, Barb Constantino, Natalie Curry, Debbie Dial, Lauren Divina, Shirley Eggan, Rob and Olivia Flack, Therese Forster, Lisa Geradi, Adam Gish, Jordan Gussin, Elmer and Etta Hamming, Karen Hanson, Aimee Hirabayashi, Marilyn Holen, Angela Horton, Jane Johnson, Natalie Johnson, Val Jones, Georgette Kinoshita, Barbara Kuznetz, Cindy Little, Dessa Lobbestael, Lisa Long, Krissy and Mike Magee, Bill Mason, Don MacInnes, Debbie Matthews, Mellody Matthes,

Gloria McCunnas, David McKoski, Cheri Myer, Kathy Meyer, Melonie Miller, Geoff Miller, Mark Neidlinger, Gary Paine, Mia Parker-Williams, Lisa Phillips, Brian and Gwyenne Poole, Tracey Potter, Mary Jo Pritza, Jasmine Riach, Sally Riewald, Barbara and John Claude Renoux, Justin Ronning, Chad Sandness, Frankie, Jochen, Andy, and Peter Snyder, Gary and Ruth, Craig and Sharon Smith, Joyce Swanson, Susan Toth, Barb Vadakin, Ed Walker, Susan Walker, Riley Wallace, Mike and Amy Watson, Jo Lynn Woods, Meg and George Wolcott, Alison Wysong, June Zacharias, Ruby, Cougar and Husky.

Whidbey Island Community:

Color Box, Freeland. Amy Cyprian and Sean Nordin. CPI Plumbing & Heating. Brandon Diers, Service Tech. Prairie Center in Coupeville. All employees, specifically Jennifer, Jeff, Claudia, Dee, Melissa, and Cindy.

Dentist Office, Seattle

Dr. Richard Green, Heather Muller, Cathy Craig, Kelli Brott, Helen Wong, Meghan Holt, Alene Wick.

Dentist Office, Oak Harbor

Dr. Valeria Cicrich, Kendra Wallace, Kina Thompson, Lisa Vanden Haak Sanchez, Summer Wentland, Mary Amuad, Naomi Dorman.

Retired Nurse:

Sue Lashley served as a nurse to me at my home and the hospital both with the brain aneurysm and APL leukemia. Daily she made a difference.

The medical personnel make a tremendous difference for others who are dealing with challenges. If they weren't there for us we would, by vast numbers, not be able to live and be with our loved ones. We can and should make efforts to thank them for helping us. All of you matter.

Doctors and Nurses, Harborview:
Started February 10, 2007
- Dr. Laligam N. Sekhar
- Dr. Nate Nare
- Ethel House, R.E.N. Assistant (Queenie)
- Zulfa Nuri, R.N.
- Katie Moore, R.N.
- Dinesh Ramanathan, Neurological Surgery
- Susan Richey, Patient Care Coordinator Neurological Surgery

Radiologists Harborview – September 24, 2010

Basavaraj Ghodke – Physician, Ryan Butler – Radiology Technician, Laura Nelson – Nurse Manager of Neuro angio, Patrice O'Heven – Radiology Technician, Mark Pickos – Radiologist Nurse, Reza Taheri – Physician.

Doctor Providence in Everett and Whidbey in Coupeville

Peter YZ Jiang, M.D., Ph.D., Hematology/Oncologist

Nurses at Providence in Everett – June 1, 2009 – June 29, 2009

Debbie (evenings), Sue (days), Darcy (nights), Chris (evenings), Brittany, Brianne, Cindy, Chanel, Kelly (CNA), Nicole (CNA), Kathy Ketchum (IV/RN/CRNI)

Emergency Room Physicians, Whidbey General Hospital:

Samir Bishai, M.D., John Plastino, M.D.

Nurses at Whidbey General Hospital – Intensive Care Unit and Medical/Surgical Unit in Coupeville – September 10, 2009 – September 29, 2009

Christie and Sarah

Whidbey Staff at MAC – July 20, 2009 – April 28, 2010

Lynette Angkaw, L.P.N., Michelle Beesley, R.N., B.S.N., CWOCN; Ann Bell, R.N., O.C.N.; Jackie Bruns, R.N., O.C.N.; Melinda Bucholz, R.N.; Susan Cary; Erin Christensen, Clerk; Laurie Davenport, L.P.N.; Dee Giordan, Clerk; Krista Gogna; Line Goulet; Diana Graham; Ginny Green, R.N.; Julie Guilbert, R.N., O.C.N.; Dana Harkins; Marta Jensen, R.N., O.C.N.; Deb Jones; Colleen Klamm, R.N.; Don Miller, R.N., O.C.N., C.D.E.; Ivee Morgan; June Peteroli, Clerk; Maria Reyes, Lead Clerk;

Dawn Sellgren, R.N.; Candy Thomas, R.N., O.C.N.; Lisa Toomey, R.N., O.C.N.; Shannon Tumblin, R.N.; Ann Weilandt, Clerk; Renee Yanke, A.R.N.P., M.S., A.O.C.N.

Whidbey Island Internal Medicine

Lee W. Roof, M.D. – 2003 to current. Jana Best, Receptionist, Sherree Castleberry, R.M.A., Tami Hunt, C.M.A., Kristen Wheeler, PA-C.

The Pulse: One Team • One Purpose • Caring for You

A Publication of Whidbey General Hospital for the Whidbey Island Community, Volume 18 Number 1 – Winter 2011 – Teresa Trebon and Trish Rose, editor. Stephanie Haskins' article and picture – Winter 2011 edition, pages 9-10.

About the Authors

Stephanie Ione Haskins

This is Stephanie's first book. The story is true. She almost died from a brain aneurysm. She was highly motivated and worked to recover. She wants to share her story with others. While working on this story she was diagnosed with APL leukemia. This became her second battle, and she was more determined than ever to share this because of how cancer affects millions of people.

She graduated from the University of Washington with an English degree, and she is still a Husky fan. She decided after working as a secretary she needed to get a teaching degree, so she got a second degree from Central Washington University. Later, she earned a Master's Degree in Education Administration from Seattle Pacific University.

She was an educational consultant, a principal, and a teacher over the course of her career. She worked as an educational consultant for Seattle, Lake Washington, and Highline School Districts. She also worked for Dr. Terry Bergeson, Superintendent of Public Instruction, at OSPI, to help schools improve student performance. She had been a principal in Seattle at Madison Middle School and N.O.M.s Middle School. She spent six years as principal at Canyon Park Jr. High in Northshore School District, and prior to that she was the first principal for the alternative schools at B.E.S.T High School, Northstar Junior High School, and Community

Elementary School in the Lake Washington School District. She had taught in the Everett School district at both Everett High School and North Middle School. She started her teaching career at the junior high in Central Kitsap School District.

To this day she loves education, especially seeing kids learn and grow. She hopes this book provides information that is both helpful and supportive to people with challenges they may meet.

Most of all, she has a new appreciation for humdingers.

Paula Lanier Seaman

This is Paula's first book. This book has been completed because of her commitment to Stephanie's recovery from the brain aneurysm and cancer.

Paula graduated from Washington State University and is an avid Coug fan to this day. She taught high school English in Japan for two years and served as a Peace Corps Volunteer in Micronesia. She moved to Chicago, received her Master's Degree in Education from DePaul University, and taught in the Chicago Public Schools for four years. She then returned to Washington State and spent four years with the Seattle Public Schools teaching 8th grade. Currently she is in her seventh year of teaching in the Oak Harbor School District and completing her administrative credentials.

She loves Whidbey Island, especially gardening, the outdoors, her dog, Ruby, and longs for a John Deere tractor of her very own.

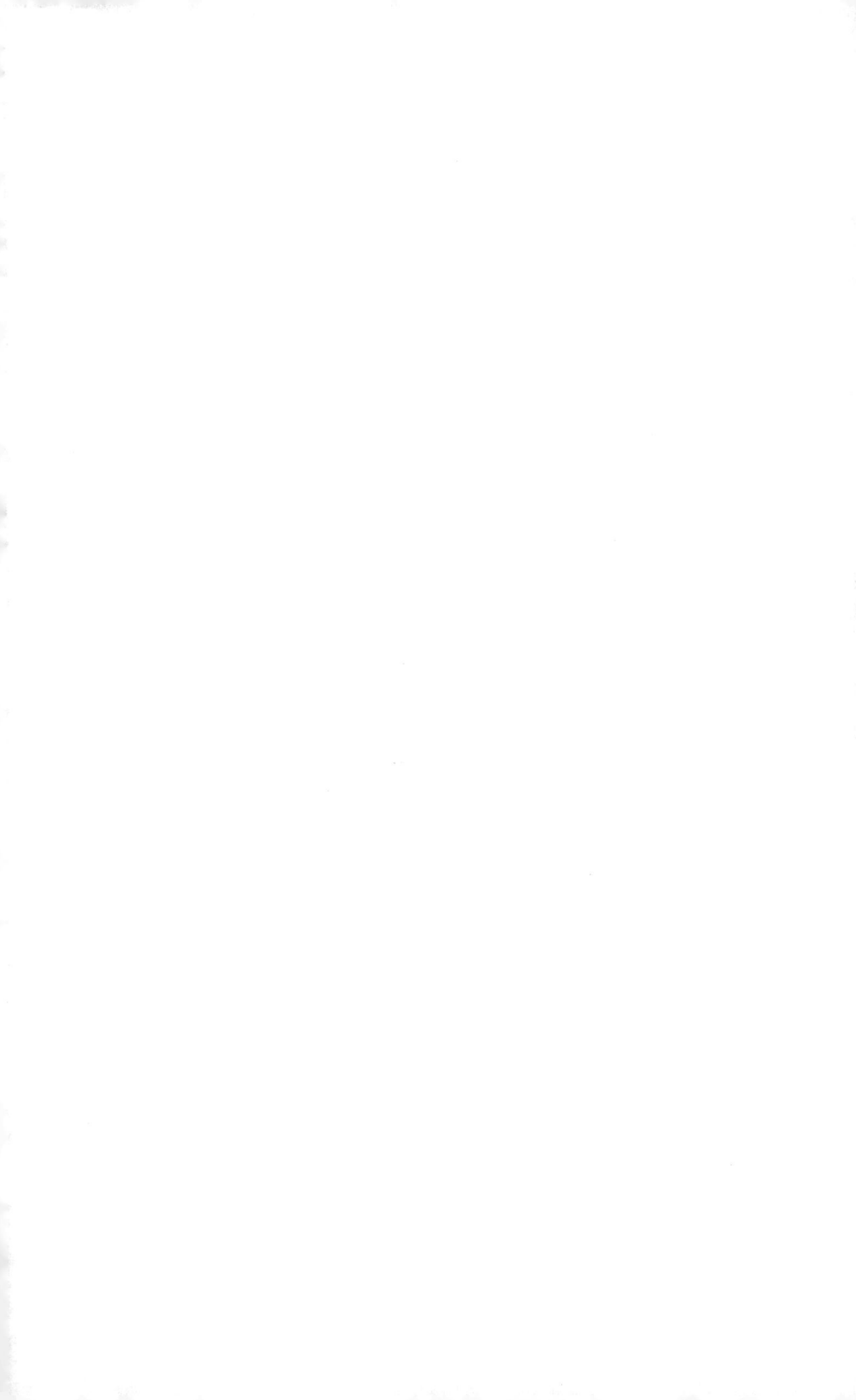

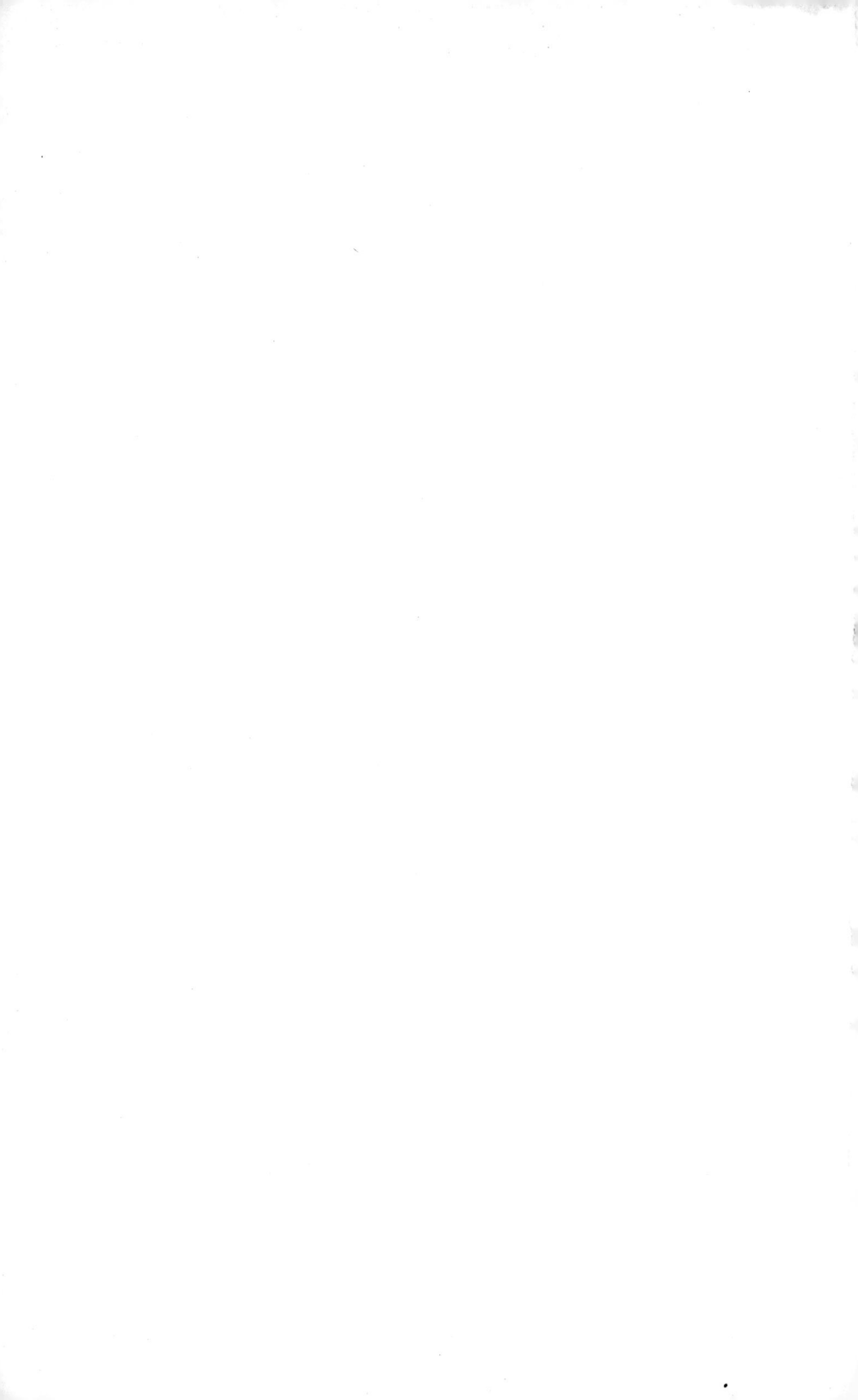